T0301704

ROC Analysis for Classification and Prediction in Practice

This book presents a unified and up-to-date introduction to ROC methodologies, covering both diagnosis (classification) and prediction. The emphasis is on the conceptual underpinning of ROC analysis and the practical implementation in diverse scientific fields. A plethora of examples accompany the methodologic discussion using standard statistical software such as R and STATA. The book arrives after two decades of intensive growth in both the methods and the applications of ROC analysis and presents a new synthesis. The authors provide a contemporary, integrated exposition of ROC methodology for both classification and prediction and include material on multiple-class ROC. This book avoids lengthy technical exposition and provides code and datasets in each chapter. *Receiver Operating Characteristic Analysis for Classification and Prediction* is intended for researchers and graduate students, but will also be useful for those that use ROC analysis in diverse disciplines such as diagnostic medicine, bioinformatics, medical physics, and perception psychology.

Chapman & Hall/CRC Biostatistics Series

Recently Published Titles

Advanced Statistics in Regulatory Critical Clinical Initiatives
Edited By Wei Zhang, Fangrong Yan, Feng Chen, Shein-Chung Chow

Medical Statistics for Cancer Studies
Trevor F. Cox

Real World Evidence in a Patient-Centric Digital Era
Edited by Kelly H. Zou, Lobna A. Salem, Amrit Ray

Data Science, AI, and Machine Learning in Pharma
Harry Yang

Model-Assisted Bayesian Designs for Dose Finding and Optimization
Methods and Applications
Ying Yuan, Ruitao Lin and J. Jack Lee

Digital Therapeutics: Strategic, Scientific, Developmental, and Regulatory Aspects
Oleksandr Sverdlov, Joris van Dam

Quantitative Methods for Precision Medicine
Pharmacogenomics in Action
Rongling Wu

Drug Development for Rare Diseases
Edited by Bo Yang, Yang Song and Yijie Zhou

Case Studies in Bayesian Methods for Biopharmaceutical CMC
Edited by Paul Faya and Tony Pourmohamad

Statistical Analytics for Health Data Science with SAS and R
Jeffrey Wilson, Ding-Geng Chen and Karl E. Peace

Design and Analysis of Pragmatic Trials
Song Zhang, Chul Ahn and Hong Zhu

ROC Analysis for Classification and Prediction in Practice
Christos Nakas, Leonidas Bantis and Constantine Gatsonis

Controlled Epidemiological Studies
Marie Reilly

Statistical Methods for Health Disparity Research
J. Sunil Rao, Ph.D.

For more information about this series, please visit: https://www.routledge.com/Chapman--Hall-CRC-Biostatistics-Series/book-series/CHBIOSTATIS

ROC Analysis for Classification and Prediction in Practice

Christos T Nakas
Leonidas E Bantis
Constantine A Gatsonis

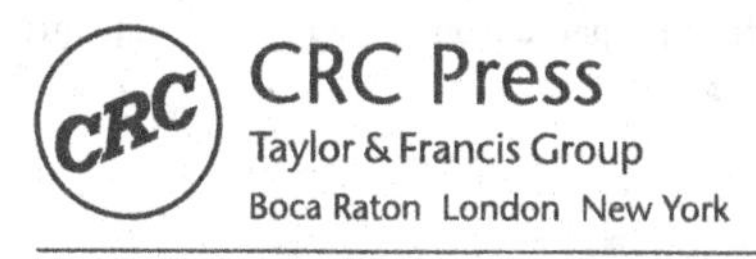

CRC Press is an imprint of the
Taylor & Francis Group, an **informa** business
A CHAPMAN & HALL BOOK

Designed cover image: © Christos T Nakas, Leonidas E Bantis and Constantine A Gatsonis

First edition published 2023
by CRC Press
6000 Broken Sound Parkway NW, Suite 300, Boca Raton, FL 33487-2742

and by CRC Press
4 Park Square, Milton Park, Abingdon, Oxon, OX14 4RN

CRC Press is an imprint of Taylor & Francis Group, LLC

ISBN: 978-1-482-23370-4 (hbk)
ISBN: 978-1-032-48022-0 (pbk)
ISBN: 978-0-429-17014-0 (ebk)

DOI: 10.1201/9780429170140

Typeset in CMR10 font
by KnowledgeWorks Global Ltd.

Publisher's note: This book has been prepared from camera-ready copy provided by the authors.

CN: Dedicated to my kids, Theo, Ellie, and Philip.
LB: Dedicated to my family.
CG: Dedicated to my students and collaborators in studies of diagnosis and prediction during the past 35 years.

Contents

Foreword xiii

Preface xv

1 Introduction 1
1.1 Diagnostic and Predictive Accuracy of Tests 1
1.2 Receiver Operating Characteristic Curve 2
1.2.1 Why ROC analysis? 4
1.3 Topics and Organization of the Book 6
1.4 Case Studies and Datasets Used 7
1.4.1 Brucellosis study 7
1.4.2 Late-onset sepsis in neonates 8
1.4.3 Pancreatic cancer markers 8
1.4.4 Parkinson disease markers 9
1.4.5 Diagnostic performance of mammography 10
1.5 Software Used in this Book 13

2 Measures of Diagnostic and Predictive Performance 17
2.1 Fundamentals 18
2.1.1 Binary tests 18
2.1.2 General formulation 22
2.2 The Receiver Operating Characteristic curve and its summaries 23
2.2.1 Definition of the ROC curve 23
2.2.2 Empirical ROC curve 24
2.2.2.1 Empirical ROC curve in the absence of ties . 25
2.2.2.2 Empirical ROC in the presence of ties 25
2.2.3 Summaries of the ROC Curve 26
2.2.3.1 Area under the ROC curve 28
2.2.3.2 Maximum of the Youden index 29
2.2.3.3 Length of the ROC curve 31
2.3 Graphs and Metrics Related to the ROC Curve 32
2.3.1 Free-Response ROC analysis (FROC) 33
2.3.2 gROC curve 33
2.3.3 Net benefit approaches and decision curve analysis . . 34
2.3.4 Predictive ROC (PROC) curve 34
2.3.5 Precision-Recall curve 36

2.4 Illustrations . . . 39
2.4.1 Continuous-scaled marker . . . 39
2.4.2 Ordinal-scaled marker . . . 42
2.4.3 Binary-scaled marker . . . 43
2.5 Exercises . . . 44

3 Statistical Inference for the ROC Curve 47
3.1 Statistical Models for the ROC Curve . . . 48
3.1.1 Binormal and other parametric models . . . 48
3.1.1.1 The Box-Cox transformation in the ROC curve context . . . 51
3.1.1.2 ROC curve estimation for the binormal model via ordinal regression: ordinal marker measurements . . . 54
3.1.1.3 ROC estimation for continuous-scaled data without distributional assumptions . . . 57
3.1.1.4 Pointwise confidence bands for ROC curves derived from continuous marker data . . . 58
3.1.2 Inference for the empirical ROC curve . . . 60
3.1.2.1 Hypothesis testing for the empirical ROC curve . . . 62
3.1.3 Nonparametric models . . . 63
3.1.3.1 Kernel-based ROCs . . . 63
3.1.3.2 Spline-based ROCs . . . 66
3.2 Inference for ROC Summary Measures . . . 70
3.2.1 Statistical inference for the AUC . . . 71
3.2.1.1 Nonparametric methods . . . 71
3.2.1.2 Parametric methods . . . 72
3.2.1.3 Bootstrap-based inference for AUC . . . 74
3.2.2 Hypothesis testing for AUC . . . 75
3.2.3 Statistical inference for the partial Area Under the ROC Curve (pAUC) . . . 77
3.2.4 Selection of optimal points and cut-offs, Youden index 78
3.2.5 Sensitivity and Specificity at specific cut-off points . . 81
3.3 Exercises . . . 83

4 Comparing ROC Curves 85
4.1 General Considerations . . . 86
4.2 Comparing ROC Curves via their AUC . . . 86
4.2.1 Parametric AUC comparisons . . . 87
4.2.1.1 Ordinal categorical test data . . . 87
4.2.1.2 Normally distributed, continuous test data . 87
4.2.1.3 Non-normally distributed, continuous test data . . . 89

4.2.1.4 Tests based on the binormal model 91
4.2.2 Nonparametric AUC comparisons 93
4.2.2.1 A general method using U-statistics 93
4.2.2.2 Bootstrap and other alternative nonparametric methods 94
4.3 Comparing ROC Curves via their Youden Index 95
4.3.1 Comparison for normally distributed marker data . . . 96
4.3.2 Comparisons without the normality assumption 98
4.3.3 Nonparametric kernel-based comparisons 98
4.3.4 Omnibus comparisons of ROC curves 100
4.3.4.1 Parametric methods for omnibus ROC curve comparisons 100
4.3.4.2 A nonparametric method for omnibus ROC curve comparisons 103
4.4 AUC-based Testing for Equivalence or Non-inferiority of Diagnostic Tests 104
4.5 Sample Size Considerations 105
4.5.1 Sample size for inference about a single AUC 106
4.5.2 Sample size for comparing two AUCs 106
4.5.3 Choice of metric for ROC comparisons 108
4.6 Exercises 109

5 The ROC Surface and k-class Classification for $k > 2$ 111
5.1 The ROC Surface for Ordered Three-class Classification . . . 112
5.1.1 The three-class model 112
5.1.2 ROC surface modelling 114
5.1.2.1 Empirical and general nonparametric estimation 114
5.1.2.2 Parametric estimation, the trinormal model . 115
5.2 The Volume Under the ROC Surface (VUS) and its Estimation 118
5.3 Hypothesis Testing for VUS 119
5.3.1 Hypothesis testing for a single VUS 119
5.3.2 Comparison of diagnostic markers via their VUS estimates 121
5.4 Hypothesis Testing for the Entire ROC Surface 122
5.4.1 Comparing two markers 122
5.4.2 Box-Cox transformation when comparing two markers 125
5.4.3 Special case: Assessment of a single marker 126
5.5 The ROC Umbrella, Different Order Restrictions 127
5.6 ROC Hypersurfaces, Multiple-class Classification 129
5.7 Generalized Youden Index, Cut-off Point Selection in Multiple-class Classification 130
5.7.1 Estimation of the generalized Youden index and respective cut-off points 131

5.7.2 Euclidean distance from the perfection corner to obtain optimized cut-offs in the 3-class setting 133
5.8 Further Topics in Three- and k-class ROC Methodology . . . 135
5.9 Exercises 136

6 ROC Regression 137
6.1 Regression Models for ROC Analysis 138
6.1.1 Parametric Methods 139
6.1.1.1 Ordinal categorical markers 139
6.1.1.2 Continuous markers 139
6.1.1.3 Computations 140
6.1.2 Semi-parametric Methods 141
6.1.2.1 Location-scale models 141
6.1.2.2 Cox regression models 142
6.1.3 Further reading 143
6.2 Optimal Prediction with Combinations of Markers 144
6.2.1 Prediction using machine learning techniques 145
6.2.2 Prediction using the binormal model 146
6.2.3 Biomarker combinations maximizing the Youden index 148
6.2.4 ROC curve evaluation after logistic regression 150
6.3 ROC Curve Analysis in Complex Designs 153
6.3.1 Analysis of correlated ordinal categorical data 153
6.3.2 Hierarchical ROC analysis 154
6.3.3 Jackknife and Bootstrap Methods 154
6.3.4 Sample size considerations 155
6.4 Time-dependent ROC Analysis 156
6.4.1 Definitions of time-dependent sensitivity and specificity 156
6.4.2 Estimation 157
6.4.3 Cumulative/dynamic 157
6.4.4 Incident/static 158
6.4.5 Incident/dynamic 159
6.5 Exercises 159

7 Missing Data and Errors-in-Variables in ROC Analysis 161
7.1 ROC Analysis under Verification Bias 161
7.1.1 Verification bias in binary test evaluation 162
7.1.1.1 Illustration using R 164
7.1.2 Verification bias in ROC curve estimation 168
7.1.3 Verification bias for three class (ROC surface) analysis 170
7.1.3.1 Implementation using R 171
7.2 Marker Measurements in the Presence of a Limit of Detection 174
7.2.1 Empirical ROC for markers with LoD 174
7.2.2 Parametric models for markers with LoD: Box-Cox and the extended generalized gamma ROC curves 175

7.2.3 A hybrid approach 177
7.3 ROC Analysis with Measurement Error 177
7.3.1 Parametric analysis for markers with measurement error 178
7.4 ROC Analysis under Imperfect Reference Standard Bias . . 179
7.4.1 Binary markers under an imperfect reference standard 180
7.4.2 Non-binary markers under an imperfect reference standard 182
7.5 Exercises 183

Bibliography **185**

Index **211**

Foreword

For those about to ROC, we salute you!

About the Authors

Christos T Nakas is Full Professor of Biometry at the University of Thessaly, Volos, Greece, and Primary Investigator/Consultant of Biostatistics and Data Science at the Department of Clinical Chemistry (UKC), Inselspital, University Hospital of the University of Bern, Bern, Switzerland.

Leonidas E Bantis is an Assistant Professor of Biostatistics at the Department of Biostatistics and Data Science, University of Kansas Medical Center, and a member of the University of Kansas Cancer Center, Kansas City, KS, USA.

Constantine A Gatsonis is *Henry Ledyard Goddard University Professor of Biostatistics*, at Brown University School of Public Health, Providence, RI, USA. He is the founding Chair of the Department of Biostatistics and founding Director of the Center for Statistical Sciences at Brown.

Preface

This book arrives at a time when ROC analysis has become a mature area of statistical methods and is used across the spectrum of subject matter studies of diagnosis and prediction. In this conjuncture we had a lot of material from which to choose and several audiences to address. We took an eclectic approach, informed by recent directions in ROC methodology and by what seemed important from our collective experience in interdisciplinary research. As such, the book is largely motivated by the paradigms of ROC analysis in the evaluation of biomarkers and imaging modalities.

We tried to balance the material between theory and implementation of ROC-related procedures in practice and included computer code using `R` and `Stata`. We emphasized the conceptual basis of ROC methods and highlighted the key attributes that inform the relevance of these methods to interdisciplinary research. And although we avoided theoretical derivations, we included a rich list of references to statistical literature for the interested readers. To help the reader digest the content, we added exercises at the end of each chapter. We hope that the book can be useful to interested graduate level students and to researchers from a wide range of disciplines and different industries.

The cornerstone of this book was laid during the XXVIIth International Biometric Conference (IBC 2014) in Florence, Italy, where two of the authors (CG and CN) met and agreed upon the main content and philosophy of the book. The following buildup occurred during the preparation of a half-semester course for the MSc in Biostatistics of the University of Zurich, Switzerland, where CN gave the course entitled "Statistical evaluation of diagnostic and predictive accuracy" during the spring semester of 2016. A significant part of the content of the book was prepared then and the feedback from the students provided useful guidance for the next steps. A bit later, LB completed the authors' team and gave the needed boost leading to delivering this final output.

Several people helped during the writing of this book. The authors are grateful and would like to acknowledge Constantin Yiannoutsos, Reinhard Furrer, Samuel Noll, Alexander Leichtle, Kosmas Sarafidis, John Dalrymple-Alford, Martin Fiedler, Eleni Verykouki, Samantha Morrison, Hemant Ishwaran, Shang-Ying Shiou, Ben Herman, Helga Marques, Xiao Hua (Andrew) Zhou, John V. Tsimikas, Qingxiang Yan, Peng Shi Kate Young, Brian Mosier and Benjamin Brewer. John Kimmel encouraged and facilitated the development of the book. David Grubbs helped bring it to a successful finish.

We sincerely hope that it will be a useful read for all those who will decide to invest their time studying it.

1

Introduction

CONTENTS

1.1 Diagnostic and Predictive Accuracy of Tests 1
1.2 Receiver Operating Characteristic Curve 2
  1.2.1 Why ROC analysis? 4
1.3 Topics and Organization of the Book 6
1.4 Case Studies and Datasets Used 7
  1.4.1 Brucellosis study 7
  1.4.2 Late-onset sepsis in neonates 8
  1.4.3 Pancreatic cancer markers 8
  1.4.4 Parkinson disease markers 9
  1.4.5 Diagnostic performance of mammography 10
1.5 Software Used in this Book 13

1.1 Diagnostic and Predictive Accuracy of Tests

In diagnostic test evaluation, the term *accuracy* is typically used to describe the degree of success in detecting the true state of a target condition (*diagnostic accuracy*) or in predicting the true state of a target condition using available test information (*predictive accuracy*). The detection task is often called *classification* in settings beyond medicine. The information used in the task of detection and prediction is obtained from the results of *tests*, which involve such modalities as devices (e.g.imaging technologies), laboratory assays (e.g. laboratory measurements or molecular biomarkers), and algorithms (e.g. risk scores in medicine or prediction rules in machine learning).

Test results can be represented by variables with discrete, continuous, or mixed distributions. For example, the result of a radiologist's interpretation of a mammogram for the detection of breast cancer may be binary (e.g. yes/no for the presence of breast cancer), ordinal categorical (e.g. normal, possibly abnormal, equivocal, probably abnormal, definitely abnormal), or continuous (e.g. probability of breast cancer) [211]. As another example, the result of a

DOI: 10.1201/9780429170140-1

Positron Emission Tomography (PET) scan of lung cancer patients is quantified via the Standard Uptake Value (SUV), a continuous variable representing the uptake of the radio-tracer in the anatomical region of interest [138]. The change in SUV values during the course of therapy can be used to assess response to therapy and/or to predict patient outcomes, such as survival.

The *target condition* may also be represented by variables with discrete, continuous, or mixed distributions. For example, arterial stenosis may be assessed by percent stenosis, which has a continuous or a mixed distribution, with the latter occurring when a fraction of the individuals assessed does not have stenosis in the particular artery. Alternatively, the degree of stenosis may be expressed as an ordinal categorical variable (none, moderate, severe) or even as a binary variable (stenosis at or below 50% vs stenosis above 50%.) [202]. In the vast majority of cases, the target condition is assumed to be binary or categorical.

The two concepts of accuracy correspond to the two conditional distributions that can be defined from the joint distribution of test results (T) and true states of the target condition (D). The accuracy of detection is assessed from the conditional distribution of T given D while the accuracy of prediction is assessed from the conditional distribution of D given T. In the common setting of a binary target condition (D=1 if the target condition is absent, D=2 if the target condition is present) and binary test result (also T=1 or 2), the diagnostic accuracy is usually measured by the *sensitivity* of the test, defined as the conditional probability $P(T = 2|D = 2)$, and the *specificity* of the test, defined as the conditional probability $P(T = 1|D = 1)$. The predictive accuracy is usually measured by the *positive predictive value* of the test, defined as the conditional probability $P(D = 2|T = 2)$ and the *negative predictive value* of the test, defined as $P(D = 1|T = 1)$. The overall (marginal) agreement of test and reference standard, defined by the probability $P(T = D)$, is called the *overall accuracy* of the test and is commonly used in some fields, such as machine learning.

We note here that terminology varies across fields. For example, in machine learning, *recall* or *true positive rate* are alternative terms for sensitivity, *true negative rate* is an alternative term for specificity, *precision* is an alternative term for positive predictive value, and *false omission rate* is an alternative term for the complement of the negative predictive value. Table 2.2 in Chapter 2 summarizes the nomenclature and the definitions of accuracy metrics.

1.2 Receiver Operating Characteristic Curve

After surveying the general framework for assessing diagnostic and predictive performance, we are ready to introduce the *Receiver Operating Characteristic* (ROC) curve, which is the central topic of this book. The typical setting for

ROC analysis involves an ordinal categorical or continuous test variable T and a binary target condition D, taking values 1 (condition absent) or 2 (condition present), as noted in the previous section. Assuming that higher values of the test variable indicate higher likelihood of the presence of the target condition, for each threshold value c of T, the test result is considered "positive" for the presence of the target condition if $T > c$ and "negative" otherwise. We can then define the *sensitivity* and *specificity* as the conditional probabilities $P(T > c|D = 2)$ and $P(T \leq c|D = 1)$, respectively.

Clearly, the sensitivity and specificity of the test depend on the positivity threshold c. In fact, as c varies over the range of possible values of T, the sensitivity and specificity of the test vary from 0 to 1. The pairs of *(sensitivity, 1-specificity)* values, obtained as c varies over the entire range of possible values of T, constitute the ROC curve for T. The choice of axes for the plot ensures that the curve starts at the point (0,0), ends at (1,1), and stays entirely within the unit square. Generalizations of the ROC curve to settings in which the target condition takes more than two values are presented in Chapter 5.

The ROC curve displays the trade-off between test sensitivity and specificity across the range of values of the threshold for test positivity. A steep rise of the curve after the (0,0) point indicates that quick gains in sensitivity can be made for small losses in specificity. The Area Under the Curve (AUC) provides an overall measure of the attainable sensitivity values as specificity varies. Higher areas indicate better diagnostic accuracy for the test. We note here that the trade-off between sensitivity and specificity constitutes a *fundamental property* of diagnostic tests, with far-reaching implications for our understanding of test accuracy. In a very real sense, the sensitivity and the specificity of the test are coupled quantities and need to be studied together even in situations in which practical interest is focused on one or the other. A typical ROC curve along with respective histograms and Cumulative Distribution Functions (CDF) plots for "positive" and "negative" measurements is shown in Figure 1.1.

Although the ROC curve was introduced as a generalization of the notion of test sensitivity and specificity and is mostly used to assess *diagnostic accuracy*, the curve can also be used to assess the strength of prediction. For example, in a logistic regression model, the binary response can be considered as the "target condition" and the estimated probability of response as the test variable. The area of the resulting ROC curve is the value of the so-called *c-statistic* for the logistic regression model [109, 253]. Another example is the construction of *time-dependent* ROC curves in which the target condition is defined by an event that will take place at a future point in time [116]. The theory of time-dependent ROC curves is discussed in Chapter 6 of the book.

We conclude this brief introduction to the ROC curve by noting that similar constructions have been proposed using the positive and negative predictive values of a test. For a test positivity threshold c, the positive predictive value (PPV) is defined as the conditional probability $P(D = 2|T > c)$ and the negative predictive value (NPV) is defined as the conditional probability

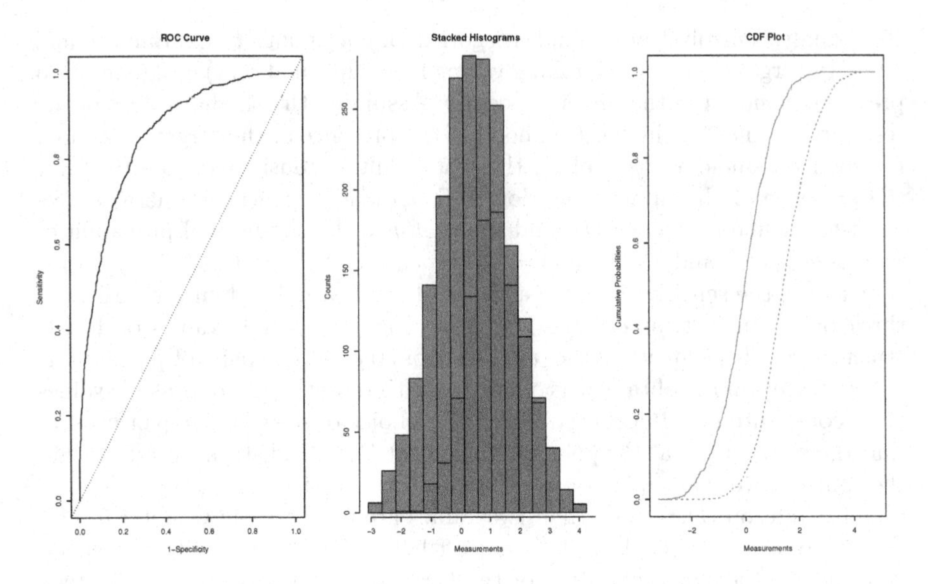

FIGURE 1.1
A typical ROC curve (left) along with respective stacked histograms (middle) and cumulative distribution functions (right) for "positive" and "negative" measurements.

$P(D = 1|T \leq c)$. The Predictive ROC curve (PROC), which is the direct analog of the ROC curve in this setting, has been discussed in the literature [242]. In addition, proposals to study the PPV and NPV separately have also appeared in the literature [179].

1.2.1 Why ROC analysis?

As discussed in the previous section, the ROC curve comprises all possible pairs of test sensitivity and specificity, derived from dichotomized test results, and measured against a binary reference standard. Thus, the curve can be understood as a generalization of the usual measures of binary test performance across the range of possible thresholds on the test. By laying bare the fundamental link between test performance and how the raw test results are interpreted as positive or negative, ROC analysis became an essential tool for test *technology assessment*. However, the utility of ROC analysis in the clinical context needs careful consideration [94].

First, it should be noted that ROC methods are used to evaluate the diagnostic and predictive performance of a marker and do not directly address patient outcomes. It is commonly understood that the effect of a test modality on patient outcomes, such as morbidity and mortality, is typically *mediated* by the therapeutic interventions taking place subsequent to a test. Thus, although the performance of a test is a key piece of information at all stages of the development of a testing modality, additional studies (such as modeling or randomized trials) are needed to address the question of how a test affects patient outcomes. To be sure, ROC analysis provides necessary information for modeling and for designing trials to evaluate patient outcomes.

Second, ROC analysis provides information that is considerably more complex than the usual estimates of binary test performance. Instead of single values of performance measures, ROC methods are used to estimate curves and derive several alternative summaries of these curves. This complexity presents a challenge to decision-makers, be they clinicians, regulators, or the general public. The most commonly used summary is the AUC, which can be interpreted as an average of test sensitivity taken over all specificity values. The AUC has simplicity on its side and also has a formal interpretation as the probability that, if a pair of subjects (one with the target condition and one without) is selected at random, the subject with the target condition will be ranked correctly by using the test.

The direct relevance of the AUC for clinical decisions has been questioned, with good reason. In many situations, only a subset of specificity or sensitivity values is of practical interest. For example, in population screening settings, high specificity values are typically of interest. However, high sensitivity values are clearly of interest in clinical settings in which a mistaken negative test result may lead to a therapy not given. To address this issue, partial AUCs have been proposed in the methodological literature but, as shown in the literature reviews, they have not achieved widespread use. Practical difficulties contribute to this reluctance to adopt the use of partial AUCs. Determining the most appropriate partial AUC for a study needs to be done in advance of the analysis to avoid serendipitous results and biased interpretations of the data. Ideally, this choice should also reflect a consensus in the field, which is specific to the particular clinical question. Thus, the simplicity of a measure that summarizes performance without the choice of a range of values of specificity or sensitivity is lost.

Single-point summaries of the ROC curve, such as the sensitivity corresponding to selected values of specificity and vice versa and optimal operating points selected to minimize cost function criteria, are also available. However, the practical utility of such single-point summaries depends on our ability to achieve particular values for test sensitivity or specificity in practice. This type of calibration is difficult for tests that require human interpretation, but it may be feasible for imaging biomarkers and laboratory tests.

The use of ROC methods to evaluate the predictive ability of markers also needs to be considered carefully, both in terms of interpretation of results and in terms of study design. Fundamentally, the ROC curve is defined and estimated conditionally on a binary reference standard. When ROC analysis is used to evaluate the performance of a predictive marker or, more generally, a predictive model, the role of binary disease status is played by the binary outcome to be predicted by the model. So the sensitivity dimension of an ROC point represents the conditional probability that the value of the marker will exceed a particular threshold given that the binary outcome will be "positive". Note that this is not the usual definition of the positive predictive value of a test, which is defined conditionally on the test result. An extension of this formulation is the so-called *time-dependent ROC* discussed in Chapter 6 of the book. In that case, the reference standard is defined by the occurrence of an event at a future time t.

Ceteris paribus, the value of sensitivity and specificity and, hence, the ROC curve is not affected by disease prevalence, while, on the contrary, the positive and negative predictive values of a test are known to depend in disease prevalence. However, as discussed in Chapters 2–4 of the book, the variance of estimated ROC parameters depends heavily on the number of subjects with *and* without the target condition and hence depends on the prevalence of the target condition.

1.3 Topics and Organization of the Book

This book discusses the theoretical underpinnings of ROC methodology and the applications of this methodology across diverse fields, from medicine to machine learning. We emphasize the conceptual basis of ROC analysis and present the statistical methods with a view toward applying these methods in various scientific domains and implementing them through software. The latter can come from the extensive collection of available packages or can be developed by the analyst. In the chapters to follow, we describe the general framework of ROC methods, discuss statistical procedures for inference, modeling, and generalization of ROC techniques, and illustrate these with applications in both standard and more complicated problems which arise in practice. We describe the entire process of analysis and implementation of these techniques using statistical software (mainly `R` and `Stata`), as well as procedures developed by the authors.

The book is organized in seven Chapters. In Chapter 1 we describe the general framework and present datasets and research projects that gave rise to questions requiring ROC methodology. In Chapter 2 we define measures of diagnostic and predictive performance of markers and explain how the ROC curve is built on the trade-off between test sensitivity and specificity, as the threshold for test positivity varies. We discuss the derivation of the empirical ROC curve for a set of data and survey how common summaries of the ROC curve, notably the AUC, is derived and interpreted.

Chapter 3 is central to the book. Here we discuss statistical inference for a single ROC curve and the corresponding indices of diagnostic accuracy. In particular, we describe parametric and non-parametric formulations of ROC analysis and discuss estimation and testing methods for summary measures of the ROC curve, notably the full and partial AUC, the Youden index, and the optimal points of the curve. Statistical methods for the comparison of ROC curves and their summary measures are discussed in Chapter 4. Design issues and sample size calculation methods are also presented therein.

In Chapter 5 we discuss the recently developed methodology for ROC analysis with three or more classes. In particular, we present the construction of the ROC surface and the calculation of its summary indices, such as the Volume Under the Surface (VUS) and the generalized Youden index. Regression methods for ROC analysis are described in Chapter 6. In the final Chapter 7, we discuss methods for ROC analysis with missing data, notably in connection with verification bias and also summarize approaches to errors-in-variables in ROC analysis.

In addition to the discussion of methods, in each chapter we present examples of applications using published data and provide computing code mainly using `R` and `Stata`. The exercises at the end of each of the following chapters are intended to help readers digest key concepts and methods.

1.4 Case Studies and Datasets Used

A variety of datasets are used throughout the book in order to illustrate methods and provide material for exercises. These datasets were derived from the authors' research in interdisciplinary collaborations. All datasets are available for download under a Creative Commons license.

1.4.1 Brucellosis study

Brucellosis is a classical intracellular granulomatous bacterial infection with worldwide distribution, especially in the developing countries. Skendros et al. (2007) [247] have studied the percentage of peripheral T-lymphocytes in brucellosis patients in order to investigate their role in disease outcome. We will be using CD3 and CD4 T-lymphocyte counts in peripheral blood for the diagnosis of brucellosis conditions, typically used in brucellosis diagnosis. The dataset (available at `http://dx.doi.org/10.13140/RG.2.2.29516.85127`) consists of 50 subjects, 35 brucellosis cases, and 15 controls. Cases can be further considered as acute (12 cases) or chronic (23 cases). Descriptive statistics are provided in Table 1.1, while boxplots for marker CD4 peripheral blood count are depicted in Figure 1.2. These data will mainly serve for illustrations of ROC methods when normality assumptions are met.

TABLE 1.1
Descriptive statistics for CD3, CD4 counts in the peripheral blood of 15 controls and 35 brucellosis cases from Skendros et al. (2007) [247]. Significance of Shapiro-Wilk normality test is also provided.

	Mean (Std. dev.)	Median (Min-Max)	SW p-value
CD3			
Controls	75.20 (5.99)	75.0 (62-85)	0.894
Cases	84.63 (8.81)	86.0 (66-98)	0.258
Acute	88.67 (6.50)	88.5 (79-98)	0.969
Chronic	82.52 (9.23)	85.0 (66-96)	0.117
CD4			
Controls	52.87 (6.97)	51.0 (42-66)	0.479
Cases	70.80 (10.14)	72.0 (49-92)	0.956
Acute	67.92 (9.34)	69.5 (49-82)	0.833
Chronic	72.30 (10.42)	74.0 (54-92)	0.841

1.4.2 Late-onset sepsis in neonates

Morbidity and mortality of nosocomial/late-onset sepsis (LOS) are high in preterm neonates. Accurate and timely diagnosis of sepsis is clinically difficult in the neonatal period. In addition, the reliability of existing diagnostic tests for early identification of septic neonates varies. Sarafidis et al. (2010) [232] have assessed the value of serum levels of soluble triggering receptor expressed on myeloid cells-1 (sTREM-1) for early diagnosis of late-onset sepsis (LOS) in neonates and compared with interleukin-6 (IL-6) which is a standard diagnostic measurement for LOS. The dataset (available at `http://dx.doi.org/10.13140/RG.2.2.22805.96482`) consists of 52 neonates of which 31 were infected (22 with confirmed sepsis, nine with possible sepsis) while 22 were non-infected. Descriptive statistics are provided in Table 1.2, while boxplots for measurements of marker sTREM-1 are depicted in Figure 1.3. These data will mainly serve for illustrations of ROC methods when normality assumptions do not hold and transformations to normality can be considered before applying ROC-related methods.

1.4.3 Pancreatic cancer markers

In a study of pancreatic cancer, Leichtle et al. (2013) [146] have collected serum samples of pancreatic carcinoma patients, controls, and pancreatitis patients and generated amino acid profiles by routine mass-spectrometry. Measurements of a series of tumor markers, such as, A1GL, A1GLP, CA19-9, etc., for 40 pancreatic cancer patients, 26 pancreatitis patients, and 40 controls were available (`http://dx.doi.org/10.13140/RG.2.2.20621.08160`). Some markers had sparse missing values. Descriptive statistics for marker CA19-9 are given in Table 1.3, while respective boxplots are depicted in Figure 1.4.

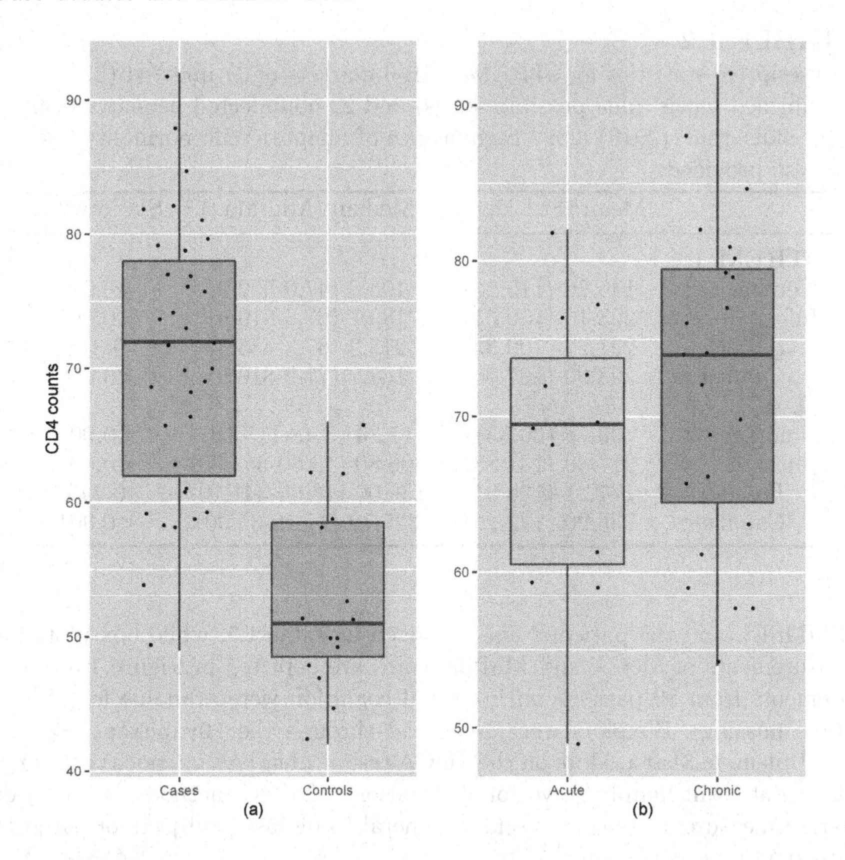

FIGURE 1.2
Boxplots of CD4 peripheral blood count. (a) Brucellosis cases vs Controls. (b) Acute cases vs Chronic cases.

Boxplots were generated through the `ggplot2` package in `R`, version 4.1.2. These data will mainly serve for illustrations of ROC surface methods in three-class classification problems.

1.4.4 Parkinson disease markers

Routine cognitive screening in Parkinson's Disease (PD) has become essential for management, to track progression and to assess clinical status in therapeutic trials. Dalrymple-Alford et al. (2010) [60] have illustrated that routinely assessing cognitive performance by using the Montreal Cognitive Assessment test (MoCA) is a valuable tool in PD screening. A total of 143 patients were examined, 83 with normal cognition, 36 with mild cognitive impairment, and 24 with dementia (`http://dx.doi.org/10.13140/RG.2.2.32452.86402`). Descriptive statistics for the MoCA test, the Mini Mental State Examination

TABLE 1.2
Descriptive statistics for sTREM-1, IL-6 markers of 31 infected (22 confirmed sepsis, nine possible sepsis) and 22 noninfected neonates from Sarafidis et al. (2010) [232]. Significance of Shapiro-Wilk normality test is also provided.

	Mean (Std. dev.)	Median (Min-Max)	SW p-value
sTREM-1			
Noninfected	145.26 (115.25)	106.8 (47.0-552.9)	<0.001
Infected	223.10 (150.61)	189.7 (67.3-810.9)	<0.001
Possible	221.24 (109.33)	213.9 (67.3-435.3)	0.818
Confirmed	223.90 (167.66)	162.7 (77.2-810.9)	<0.001
IL-6			
Noninfected	36.78 (36.35)	17.84 (3.48-115.10)	<0.001
Infected	217.80 (131.83)	306.80 (13.60-355.00)	<0.001
Possible	177.21 (128.91)	139.00 (13.60-341.10)	0.243
Confirmed	235.20 (132.26)	325.70 (17.19-35.00)	<0.001

(S-MMSE), and the patients' age are given in Table 1.5, while box plots for measurements of MoCA and MMSE scores are depicted in Figure 1.5. Measurements from 80 patients with normal cognition were available for MoCA (three missing). Boxplots were generated through the `'Graphics --> Box plot'` menu in `Stata`. More on the MoCA test at `http://www.mocatest.org`. These data will mainly serve for illustrations of ROC methods when lower marker measurements correspond in general to diseased subjects or subjects with the target condition.

1.4.5 Diagnostic performance of mammography

Full-field digital mammography (FFDM) is an established imaging modality for routine screening for breast cancer. An important contributor to the widespread adoption of FFDM was the Digital Mammography Imaging Screening Trial (DMIST) which compared the accuracy of digital and screen-film mammography in a cohort of 49,528 women who were asymptomatic for breast cancer [211]. A paired design was used in this multi-center study, according to which each participant underwent both screen-film and digital mammography in random order and was then followed up for up to two years. The reference standard was determined on the basis of results from biopsies or a follow-up mammogram. In particular, study participants were classified as positive for cancer if there was pathologic verification of breast cancer within 15 months after the initial mammogram. Participants were classified as negative for cancer if they had negative pathology findings or had a normal follow-up mammogram done at least 10 months after the initial mammogram. The DMIST study concluded that the accuracy of digital and film

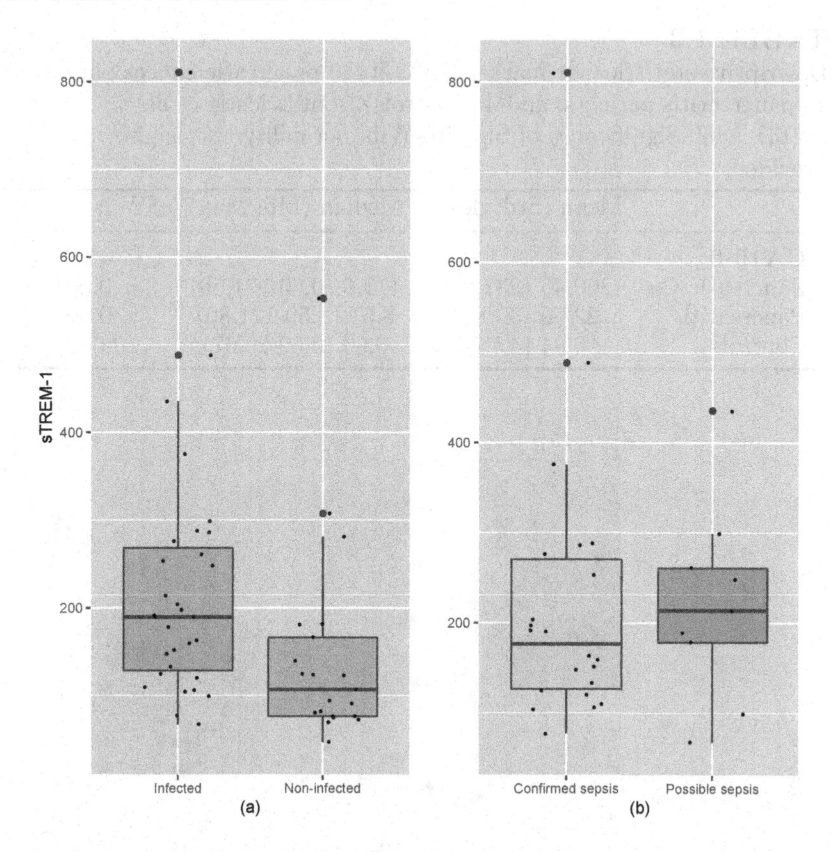

FIGURE 1.3
Boxplots along with jittered dots of sTREM-1 measurements. (a) Sepsis vs No-sepsis. (b) Confirmed sepsis vs Possible sepsis.

mammography, as measured by the area under the ROC curve, was similar between the two modalities. However, FFDM had an advantage in the subsets of women under the age of 50, who were pre- or perimenopausal, or who had mammographically dense breasts. The full data set from the trial is available to interested researchers.

The DMIST primary findings were based on the interpretations of mammograms at the participating sites, which were done by different radiologists for each modality and without knowledge of the results of the other modality. FFDM machines from four different manufacturers were used in DMIST, namely, Fischer, Fuji, General Electric, and Hologic. The number of participants differed across machines and so did the number of cancers found in these women. The scans and clinical data from DMIST were used in subsequent retrospective reader studies, which addressed more detailed questions such as the performance of FFDM for each machine manufacturer and the

TABLE 1.3
Descriptive statistics for marker CA19-9 (40 pancreatic cancer patients, 23 pancreatitis patients, and 40 controls) from Leichtle et al. (2013) [146]. Significance of Shapiro-Wilk normality test is also provided.

	Mean (Std. dev.)	Median (Min-Max)	SW p-value
CA19-9			
Pancreatic Ca	200.46 (237.85)	111.6 (0.60-971.50)	< 0.001
Pancreatitis	22.50 (30.88)	8.51 (2.50-121.80)	< 0.001
Controls	6.94 (4.74)	6.60 (0.60-20.67)	0.002

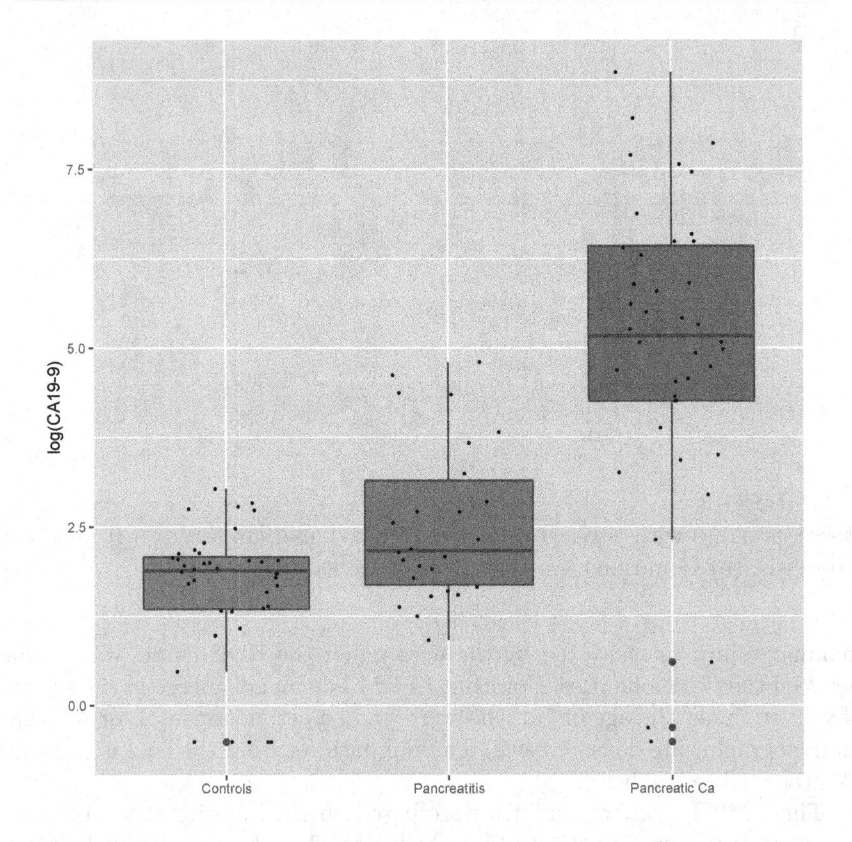

FIGURE 1.4
Boxplots of pancreatic cancer marker CA19-9 in natural log scale.

variability across test interpreters. In the largest of these reader studies, separate subsets of women with and without cancer were selected for each manufacturer and groups of radiologists interpreted the digital and screen-film scans for each woman [212]. The sample sizes for each machine type and the number of scan interpreters ("readers") is described in Table 1.5. Readings

TABLE 1.4
Descriptive statistics for MoCA, S-MMSE, and patients aged 143 Parkinson's Disease cases (83 with normal cognition (PD-N), 36 with mild cognitive impairment (PD-MCI), and 24 with dementia (PD-D)) from Dalrymple-Alford et al. (2010) [60]. Significance of Shapiro-Wilk normality test is also provided.

	Mean (Std. dev.)	Median (Min-Max)	SW p-value
MoCA			
PD-N	26.79 (2.07)	27 (22-30)	0.441
PD-MCI	23.58 (2.80)	24 (18-29)	0.918
PD-D	17.33 (4.20)	18 (10-23)	0.242
S-MMSE			
PD-N	28.18 (1.73)	29 (23-30)	<0.001
PD-MCI	25.94 (2.35)	26 (20-30)	0.249
PD-D	22.92 (2.84)	23 (17-27)	0.933
Age			
PD-N	65.13 (7.95)	66 (45-80)	0.017
PD-MCI	70.11 (8.31)	71 (42-80)	<0.001
PD-D	72.88 (7.14)	72 (59-84)	0.738

were done in random order, with a 6-week "washout" period between them in order to minimize recall. The radiologists recorded their degree of suspicion about the presence of cancer using a 7-point ordinal categorical scale. The verbal descriptors of each category were

1. The finding is definitely not malignant.
2. The finding is almost certainly not malignant.
3. The finding is probably not malignant.
4. The finding is possibly malignant.
5. The finding is probably malignant.
6. The finding is almost certainly malignant.
7. The finding is definitely malignant

These data will serve for illustrations of ROC methods when markers are ordinal-scaled.

1.5 Software Used in this Book

An important goal of this book is to introduce the reader to statistical computing to support the implementation of the methods discussed in each chapter.

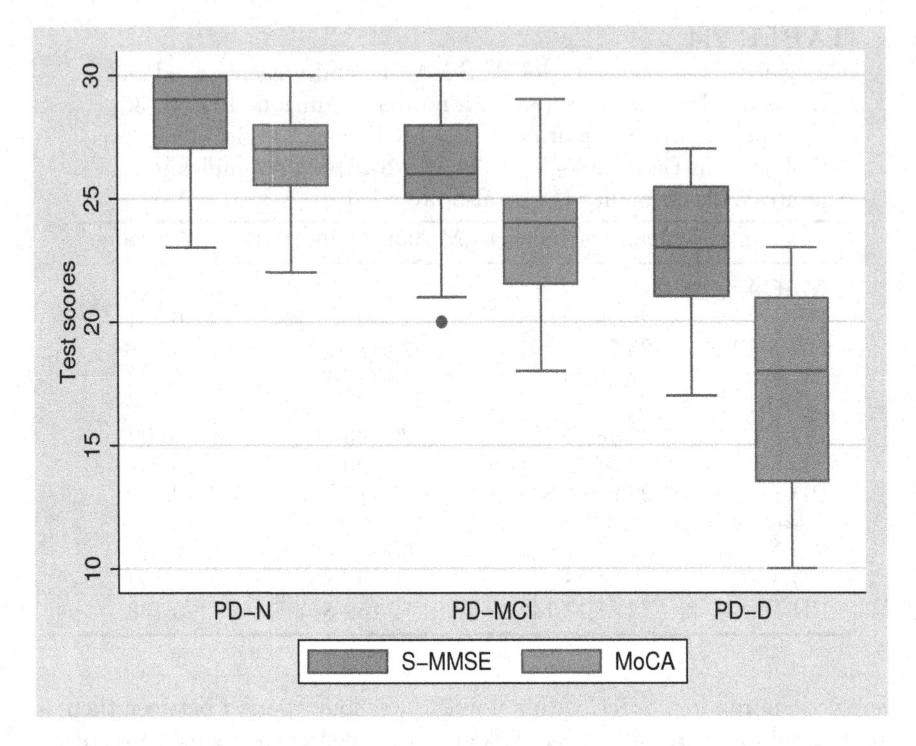

FIGURE 1.5
Boxplots of MoCA, S-MMSE scores for Parkinson's disease patients.

TABLE 1.5
Numbers of cases and interpreters by mammography machine manufacturer.

Manufacturer	Total cases	With cancer	Without cancer	Interpreters
Fischer	115	42	73	6
Fuji	98	27	71	12
GE	120	48	72	12
Hologic	28	6	22	12

In particular, we rely on subroutines from of `R`, using vesion 4.1.2 (The R Foundation for Statistical Computing, Vienna, Austria) which can be downloaded for free from `http://cran.r-project.org`, and from `Stata` 17.0 (StataCorp LLC, College Station, TX, USA), a proprietary software with a wide range of ROC-related procedures. These will be used interchangeably throughout the book with emphasis on subroutines from `R`. A wide range of alternative proprietary software choices exist with ROC analysis features, such as `MedCalc` and `SAS` among others. Similarly, open-source options include the use of `Python` and `Julia` libraries. The choice of particular software for analysis will naturally depend on availability of subroutines relevant to the scientific question.

R is freely available, and it is currently probably the most widely used software in the scientific community when it comes to the development of novel statistical techniques and their implementation. R packages exist for most of the up-to-date sophisticated methods that are developed through scientific research. Stata is a widely used proprietary software that provides a wide variety of ROC-related subroutines that can be readily implemented. Authors of this book have also used MATLAB (Mathworks Inc, Natick, MA) for various methodological developments in their published research. Most of the relevant MATLAB and R code are available on leobantis.net.

2

Measures of Diagnostic and Predictive Performance

CONTENTS

2.1 Fundamentals 18
 2.1.1 Binary tests 18
 2.1.2 General formulation 22
2.2 The Receiver Operating Characteristic curve and its summaries 23
 2.2.1 Definition of the ROC curve 23
 2.2.2 Empirical ROC curve 24
  2.2.2.1 Empirical ROC curve in the absence of ties . 25
  2.2.2.2 Empirical ROC in the presence of ties 25
 2.2.3 Summaries of the ROC Curve 26
  2.2.3.1 Area under the ROC curve 28
  2.2.3.2 Maximum of the Youden index 29
  2.2.3.3 Length of the ROC curve 31
2.3 Graphs and Metrics Related to the ROC Curve 32
 2.3.1 Free-Response ROC analysis (FROC) 33
 2.3.2 gROC curve 33
 2.3.3 Net benefit approaches and decision curve analysis 34
 2.3.4 Predictive ROC (PROC) curve 34
 2.3.5 Precision-Recall curve 36
2.4 Illustrations 39
 2.4.1 Continuous-scaled marker 39
 2.4.2 Ordinal-scaled marker 42
 2.4.3 Binary-scaled marker 43
2.5 Exercises 44

DOI: 10.1201/9780429170140-2

2.1 Fundamentals

2.1.1 Binary tests

As discussed in the previous chapter, the fundamental quantities for the evaluation of the performance of a marker (test) are, T, the value of the marker (test result), and D, the variable describing the reference information about the presence of the target condition. Throughout the book we will refer to "test" and "marker" values interchangeably. The distribution of both T and D can be discrete, continuous, or mixed. In the medical setting, T typically takes binary, ordinal categorical, or continuous values, and D takes binary values. Performance of a test is characterized by its diagnostic and its predictive performance. The *diagnostic* performance of a test is measured by quantities that are conditional on the reference standard D, such as sensitivity and specificity. The *predictive* performance is measured by quantities that are conditional on test result, such as the positive and negative predictive values.

In this chapter, we discuss several measures of diagnostic and predictive performance, beginning with the simple setting of a binary T and a binary D. In this setting, the joint distribution of the pair of test results and reference standard values is typically described by the well-known 2×2 table, in which 2 indicates the presence of the target condition ("positive" result) and 1 indicates its absence ("negative" result).

Table 2.1 represents the possible binary diagnostic test versus disease presence outcomes in a 2×2 table representation. True Negative and False Positive Fractions are complementary proportions for the non-diseased population, while True Positive and False Negative Fractions are the respective proportions for the diseased population. The words "fraction" and "rate" are used interchangeably in the ROC literature.

Note: In the medical literature, "negative" values are typically denoted by 0 and "positive" values are typically denoted by 1. In this book we adopt the 1, 2 notation, which is used broadly in the classification literature and will be useful in the sequel for simplifying further notation.

It should be noted at the outset that a binary test result is typically the outcome of dichotomizing a more complex measurement or assessment from

TABLE 2.1
Cross classification of binary test results and reference standard.

T	D		
	1	2	
1	True Negative (TN)	False Negative (FN)	Test Negative
2	False Positive (FP)	True Positive (TP)	Test Positive
	Disease Negative	Disease Positive	

an interpreter. By "interpreter" in this book, we mean human interpreters or computer software performing diagnostic tasks. The latter can be rules-based or deep-learning systems. We discuss methods for the assessment of tests with ordinal categorical or continuous outcomes later on in this chapter. Similarly, a binary target condition is often the outcome of dichotomizing a more complex reality, such as disease severity.

However, the binary model for the test and the target condition is commonly used in medicine and other areas, being useful in practice for decision-making purposes. In this binary setting, the two common measures of the *diagnostic performance* of a test characterize the test's ability to *detect* the presence or absence of the target condition. Specifically,

- the *sensitivity* of the test, defined as $P(T = 2|D = 2)$, is the conditional probability of a positive test result given that target condition is present, and
- the *specificity* of the test, defined as $P(T = 1|D = 1)$, is the conditional probability of a negative test result given that target condition is absent.

Also, the two common measures of the *predictive performance* of the test are

- the *positive predictive value (PPV)* of the test, defined as $P(D = 2|T = 2)$, that is, the conditional probability that target condition is present given that the test result was positive,
- and the *negative predictive value (NPV)* of the test, defined as $P(D = 1|T = 1)$, that is, the conditional probability that target condition is absent, given that the test result was negative.

In the language of statistical machine learning, both the detection and prediction tasks are included among *classification* techniques, as long as the reference standard variable D takes a finite number of values. The table showing test results and reference standard is called the *confusion matrix*.

Several measures of the performance of binary tests have been used across diverse scientific fields, sometimes under different names. We summarize the most commonly used measures and names in Table 2.2. The reader will note that measures of diagnostic and predictive accuracy in the table are defined as conditional probabilities or functions of conditional probabilities, with the exception of *(overall) accuracy* and *error rate*,which are defined as unconditional probabilities.

Note that F score is the harmonic mean of Sensitivity and PPV and is intended as a measure of performance that combines detection and prediction. The F_1 version of the score weighs the two components equally. A weighted version of the score, defined as $F_\beta = \frac{(1+\beta^2)\times Sens \times PPV}{\beta^2 \times Sens + PPV}$, is also used in machine learning.

TABLE 2.2
Measures of diagnostic and predictive accuracy of binary tests.

Measure names	Task	Definition
Sensitivity, True Positive Rate, Recall	Detection	$Sens = P(T = 2 \mid D = 2)$
Specificity, True Negative Rate	Detection	$Spec = P(T = 1 \mid D = 1)$
Positive Likelihood Ratio	Detection	$LR(+) = \frac{P(T=2 \mid D=2)}{P(T=2 \mid D=1)}$
Negative Likelihood Ratio	Detection	$LR(-) = \frac{P(T=1 \mid D=2)}{P(T=1 \mid D=1)}$
Odds Ratio	Detection/ Prediction	$OR = \frac{P(T=2,D=2) \cdot P(T=1,D=1)}{P(T=2,D=1) \cdot P(T=1,D=2)}$
Diagnostic Odds Ratio	Detection/ Prediction	$DOR = \frac{LR(+)}{LR(-)}$
Positive Predictive Value, Precision	Prediction	$PPV = P(D = 2 \mid T = 2)$
Negative Predictive Value	Prediction	$NPV = P(D = 1 \mid T = 1)$
False Discovery Rate	Prediction	$FDR = P(D = 1 \mid T = 2)$
False Nondiscovery Rate	Prediction	$FNDR = P(D = 2 \mid T = 1)$
Overall Accuracy		$P(D = T)$
Risk, Error rate		$P(D \neq T)$
F score , F_1 score		$F_1 = 2 \cdot \frac{Sens \times PPV}{Sens + PPV}$

Using the above definitions and Bayes Theorem, relations between the measures in Table 2.2 can be derived. For example, the likelihood ratio can be expressed as a function of sensitivity and specificity. In particular,

$$LR(+) = \frac{Sens}{1 - Spec}$$

and

$$LR(-) = \frac{1 - Sens}{Spec}.$$

Also

$$PPV = \frac{P(D = 2)Sens}{[P(D = 2)Sens + P(D = 1)(1 - Spec)]}$$

TABLE 2.3
Confusion matrix of frequencies for binary tests.

T	D		Total
	1	2	
1	n_{11}	n_{12}	n_{1+}
2	n_{21}	n_{22}	n_{2+}
Total	n_{+1}	n_{+2}	n

and similarly for the NPV,

$$NPV = \frac{P(D=1)Spec}{[P(D=1)Spec + P(D=2)(1-Sens)]}.$$

The quantity $P(D = 2)$ is commonly called the *prevalence* of the target condition, while $P(D = 1)$ is the complement of the prevalence, or $P(D = 2) = 1 - P(D = 1)$.

When the values of the test and the reference standard are available for each of n participants (units) in a study, the corresponding 2×2 table (confusion matrix) takes the form of Table 2.3.

Point estimates and confidence intervals for the measures in Table 2.2 can be readily developed using the data in Table 2.3, taking into account the design of the study generating the data. Assuming that the numbers of positives and negatives, as classified by the reference standard, to be fixed by design, the sensitivity and specificity can be derived using the common binomial distribution theory. For example, sensitivity can be estimated by $\hat{Sens} = \frac{n_{22}}{n_{+2}}$ and confidence intervals based on the binomial distribution (e.g. Wald, Wilson, exact) can be derived [41].

The well-known Wald 95% confidence interval for sensitivity is given by,

$$\left(\hat{Sens} - 1.96 \cdot \sqrt{\frac{\hat{Sens} \cdot (1-\hat{Sens})}{n_{+2}}}, \hat{Sens} + 1.96 \cdot \sqrt{\frac{\hat{Sens} \cdot (1-\hat{Sens})}{n_{+2}}}\right) \quad (2.1)$$

and similarly for specificity. However, the construction of confidence intervals for PPV and NPV typically needs to account for the fact that the denominator of their estimates is a random quantity and not fixed by the design of the study. The construction of more elaborate, simultaneous confidence intervals for sensitivity and specificity is discussed in Section 3.2.5.

Estimates of PPV, NPV can be obtained directly from the observed confusion matrix. However, as stated above, their interpretation has to take into account the design of the study. In a prospective cohort study, in which participants are enrolled on the basis of a clinical presentation with test results and reference standard information obtained prospectively, the empirical estimates of PPV and NPV would be valid and generalizable to populations with similar characteristics such as similar prevalence of disease. However, in a retrospective study in which disease status is fixed by design, the estimates of predictive values may not be generalizable.

Conditioning on test results, PPV and NPV are binomial proportions and as such, calculation of confidence intervals based on their estimates is conducted in the same way as for sensitivity and specificity. However, without conditioning on the test results, the derivation of confidence intervals needs to account for the statistical uncertainty in the denominators. A similar consideration applies to estimates of sensitivity and specificity from studies in which it is not reasonable to assume the number of diseased and non-diseased units as fixed by design [291].

2.1.2 General formulation

In most realistic settings, binary values of a test are obtained by dichotomising an underlying scale, which can be an ordinal categorical, count, or continuous variable. Examples include the 7-point ordinal categorical scale used in the DMIST trial of mammography (Section 1.4.5), the CD4 counts in the brucellosis study (Section 1.4.1) and the continuous scale for the tumor marker in the pancreatic carcinoma trial (Section 1.4.3), respectively.

The general setting of detection (a two-class classification problem) can be described as follows for a study in which a diagnostic test (marker) result is obtained on $n = n_1+n_2$ participants (units), of which n_1 does not have the target condition and n_2 has the target condition. We denote by $X_{11}, X_{12}, \ldots, X_{1n_1}$ the marker values of the group without the target condition ("non-diseased"). We assume that each X_{1i} is a value of a random variable with distribution F_1. Also we denote by $X_{21}, X_{22}, \ldots, X_{2n_2}$ the marker values of the group with the target condition ("diseased"), with distribution F_2.

The diagnostic performance of the test will depend on the amount of overlap between the two distributions, F_1 and F_2. In the rare case when these distributions do not overlap, the marker would be able to classify study participants perfectly. However, in a typical situation, there is overlap between the two distributions and marker values in the presence of the target condition tend to be larger (or smaller) than those in the absence of the target condition.

Without loss of generality, we will assume that larger values of the marker are more indicative of the presence of the target condition. Under this assumption, a "positive" test result, indicating presence of the target condition, can be defined via a *threshold (cut-off point)* value c. For threshold c, we can define the sensitivity and specificity of the test as in Section 2.1.1. In particular, the sensitivity of the diagnostic test for the threshold c is the probability that a diseased subject will be correctly classified as diseased using this threshold.

Formally,

$$Sens(c) = P(X_2 > c) = 1 - F_2(c). \tag{2.2}$$

The sensitivity can be estimated empirically by the proportion of X_2 values that are larger than c, or

$$\hat{Sens}(c) = \frac{\Sigma_{i=1}^{n_2} I(X_{2i} > c)}{n_2}. \tag{2.3}$$

Here $I(.)$ is the indicator function, i.e. $I(X_{2i} > c)$ is equal to one if $X_{2i} > c$ is true and zero otherwise, for each $i = 1, 2, \ldots, n_1$.

Similarly, the specificity of the diagnostic test for threshold c is the probability that a non-diseased subject will be correctly classified as non-diseased. Formally,

$$Spec(c) = P(X_1 \leq c) = F_1(c). \tag{2.4}$$

This quantity can be estimated empirically by the proportion of X_1 values that are at most c, or

$$\hat{Spec}(c) = \frac{\Sigma_{j=1}^{n_1} I(X_{1j} \leq c)}{n_1}. \tag{2.5}$$

2.2 The Receiver Operating Characteristic curve and its summaries

We now discuss the definition of the Receiver Operating Characteristic (ROC) curve and the summaries of diagnostic performance derived from the curve. The most common such summary is the area under the ROC curve (AUC). The discussion concentrates on curves for non-binary markers (tests). ROC curves for binary-scaled markers can also be constructed but they are rather trivial and not really useful in practice.

2.2.1 Definition of the ROC curve

As noted above, the dependence of sensitivity and specificity on the threshold used to define a "positive" test result introduces a trade-off between these two measures of diagnostic performance and indicates that the assessment of such performance needs to consider the paired values of these measures. This pairing is shown by the ROC curve, which consists of the pairs of sensitivity and 1-specificity for all possible threshold values. Formally,

$$ROC(c) = (1 - Spec(c), Sens(c)) = (1 - F_1(c), 1 - F_2(c)), c \in (-\infty, \infty).$$

The reader would note that $1 - F_1(c) = S_1(c)$ is the survival function of the test values in the non-diseased cohort, and similarly $1 - F_2(c) = S_2(c)$ is the survival function of the test values in the diseased cohort. This observation has given rise to an equivalent definition of the ROC curve as $ROC(c) = (S_1(c), S_2(c)), c \in (-\infty, \infty)$.

The ROC curve is presented graphically as a curve in the unit square, $[0,1] \times [0,1]$. Its functional form is,

$$ROC(t) = 1 - F_2(F_1^{-1}(1-t)) = S_2(S_1^{-1}(t)), t \in [0,1]. \tag{2.6}$$

F_1^{-1} is the inverse cumulative distribution function (ICDF) of F_1. The ICDF gives the marker value associated with a specific cumulative probability.

The ROC curve depicts the trade-off between sensitivity and specificity as the cut-off point used for declaring a positive test result varies between the minimum and maximum possible values of the marker. The pattern of the curve provides a detailed account of the diagnostic accuracy of the marker across all possible threshold values. In particular, desirable performance of a marker corresponds to a curve which shows a quick gain in sensitivity for a modest trade-off in specificity. The ideal point would be (0, 1) in the unit square, corresponding to a sensitivity and a specificity equal to one. A curve which stays close to the main diagonal of the unit square would indicate relatively poor diagnostic performance for a marker.

For theoretical and practical reasons, a monotone trade-off between sensitivity and specificity would be desirable. Such a pattern corresponds to a *concave* ROC curve and defines the class of *proper* ROC curves. We discuss proper ROC curves again in Section 2.2.3.3.

2.2.2 Empirical ROC curve

Empirical estimators of the ROC curve can be readily obtained from the available marker values. Using the notation established earlier in this chapter, the data set consists of marker values $X_{11}, X_{12}, \ldots, X_{1n_1}$ for the units with the target condition ("diseased") and $X_{21}, X_{22}, \ldots, X_{2n_2}$, for the units without the target condition ("non-diseased").

Estimates of sensitivity and specificity can be obtained using formulas in Equations (2.3) and (2.5), with the threshold c ranging over all the observed data points in each group. Assuming no ties in the data, it can be easily seen that exactly $(n_1 + n_2 + 1)$ different pairs of sensitivity and specificity can be defined using the estimators $\hat{Sens}(c)$ and $\hat{Spec}(c)$. These include the $(n_1 + n_2)$ pairs corresponding to the observed cut-off points and the pair (0, 0), which would be obtained when the cut-off point is greater than the maximum of the observed values. Connecting these points with linear segments produces the empirical ROC curve.

The empirical ROC curve is a commonly used estimator of the theoretical (true) ROC curve of a marker. Model-based methods for the estimation of the ROC curve are discussed in Chapter 3. Before proceeding to a discussion of the various quantities that are used to summarize the information in an ROC curve, we present two simple examples of how empirical curves can be estimated and plotted in ROC space.

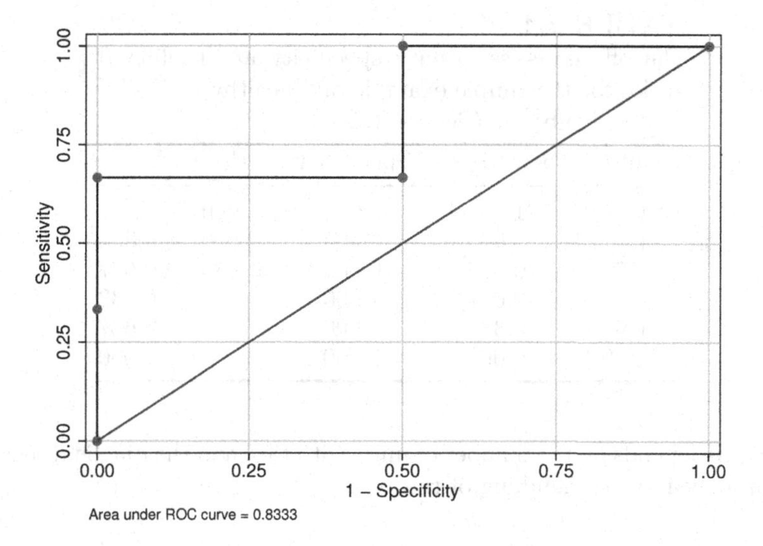

FIGURE 2.1
The ROC curve corresponding to the simple example with 2 healthy vs. 3 diseased subjects (Section 2.2.2.1), using the `roctab` command in `Stata`.

2.2.2.1 Empirical ROC curve in the absence of ties

A simple illustration of the empirical ROC curve is shown in shown in Figure 2.1. The curve was constructed using data from hypothetical groups of 2 healthy and 3 diseased units, with marker values $X_{11} = 5, X_{12} = 7$ and $X_{21} = 6, X_{22} = 8, X_{23} = 9$, respectively. Because there are no ties in these data, there are five different relevant values of the cut-off point c for the construction of the curve. Any value of c greater than 9 will result in a sensitivity estimate of zero and specificity estimate of one. Table 2.4 contains all relevant cut-off points and their respective sensitivity, specificity, and likelihood ratios, while Figure 2.1 depicts the corresponding ROC curve.

2.2.2.2 Empirical ROC in the presence of ties

Ties occur frequently when the marker takes values on an ordinal-categorical scale, such as the 7-point mammography interpreter responses in Section 1.4.5, but can also occur when the marker takes values on a continuous scale. The definition of the empirical curve is the same as before. For an illustrative example, we consider a marker taking values in five ordered categories, labeled 1 through 5. The categorical values for the non-diseased units are $\{1, 1, 2, 2, 2, 2, 3, 4\}$, while for diseased units they are $\{3, 3, 4, 4, 4, 5, 5, 5\}$. The observed values (frequencies) are shown in Table 2.5, the pairs of estimated points in Table 2.6, and the full graph in Figure 2.2. The size of increments in

TABLE 2.4
Cut-off points, sensitivity, specificity, and likelihood ratios for the simple example of 2 healthy vs. 3 diseased subjects (Section 2.2.2.1).

Cut-off	Sensitivity	Specificity	$LR(+)$	$LR(-)$
(5)	1.000	0.000	1.000	
(6)	1.000	0.500	2.000	0.000
(7)	0.667	0.500	1.333	0.667
(8)	0.667	1.000		0.333
(9)	0.333	1.000		0.667
(>9)	0.000	1.000		1.000

the curve depends on the number of units with ties, and the diagonal segments are produced by the handling of ties.

2.2.3 Summaries of the ROC Curve

The ROC curve consists of all possible values of sensitivity and 1-specificity of the marker and, in this sense, presents an extensive amount of information about marker behavior. Figure 2.3 illustrates three different scenarios of overlap between measurements of a hypothetical diagnostic marker of controls vs. cases. Histograms of marker measurements are depicted in the top row while the respective ROC curves are given in the bottom row. For scenario (a), there is nearly complete overlap between measurements of controls and cases. As a result, the respective ROC curve is very close to the main diagonal. It follows that $sens(c) \approx 1 - spec(c)$ for all c. This marker is not useful in practice. Scenario (b) presents an intermediate case which is most common in practice in this setting. There is some overlap between measurements from the two classes. This marker can be useful for diagnostic purposes. Finally, in scenario (c), there is almost perfect separation of measurements from the two classes. The latter corresponds to a nearly perfect diagnostic marker.

In practice, *summary* measures derived from the curve are used to interpret curves and compare markers. Some of these summaries, notably the full and

TABLE 2.5
Contingency table for a marker with ordinal categorical values, classified by true disease state. Numbers represent frequencies.

	1	2	3	4	5
D_1	2	4	1	1	0
D_2	0	0	2	3	3

TABLE 2.6
Cut-off points, sensitivity, specificity, and likelihood ratios for the simple example of 8 healthy vs. 8 diseased subjects (Section 2.2.2.2).

Cut-off	Sensitivity	Specificity	$LR(+)$	$LR(-)$
(1)	1.000	0.000	1.000	
(2)	1.000	0.250	1.333	0.000
(3)	1.000	0.750	4.000	0.000
(4)	0.750	0.875	6.000	0.286
(5)	0.375	1.000		0.625
(>5)	0.000	1.000		1.000

the partial area under the ROC curve, characterize the *average* of True Positive Rate values over a range of False Positive Rate values. Other summaries characterize the curve at specific points, such as the value of sensitivity corresponding to a specificity value of practical interest and conversely, or points satisfying specific optimality criteria. For example, a commonly used quantity is the maximum distance from the curve to the main diagonal of the unit square. This measure is equivalent to the maximum of the Youden index that will be described in Section 2.2.3.2.

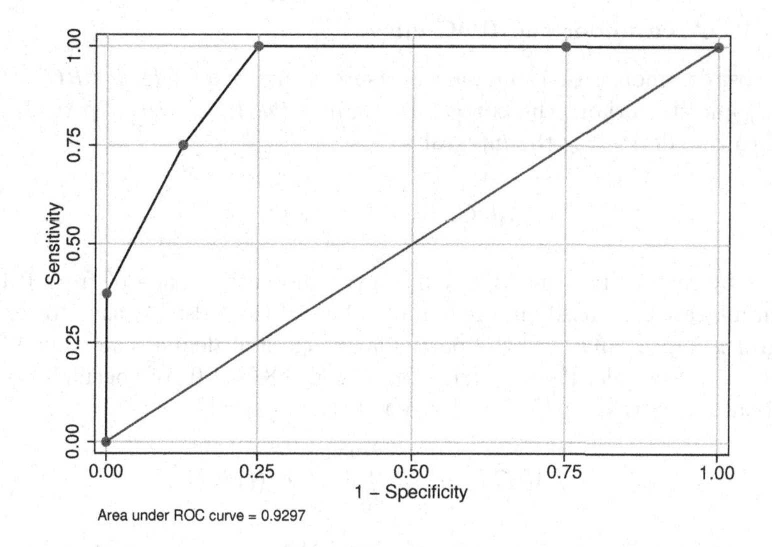

FIGURE 2.2
The ROC curve corresponding to the simple example with eight healthy vs. eight diseased subjects (Section 2.2.2.2), using the `roctab` command in Stata.

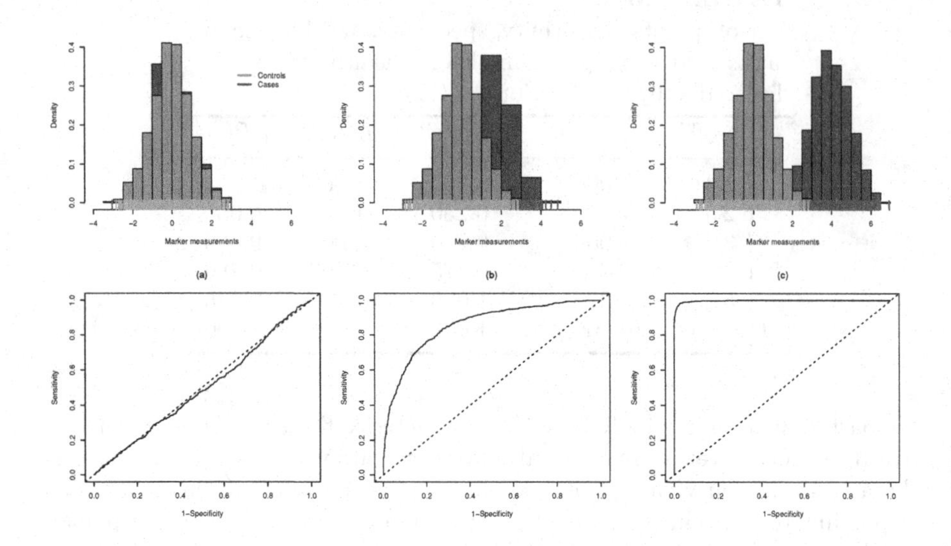

FIGURE 2.3
Histograms (first row) and respective ROC curves (second row) for three cases of hypothesized marker measurements.

2.2.3.1 Area under the ROC curve

The most commonly used summary measure is the *Area Under the ROC Curve* (AUC) and its variant, the *partial Area under the ROC Curve* (pAUC). The AUC can be derived as the integral

$$AUC = \int_0^1 ROC(t)dt, \tag{2.7}$$

that is by integrating the ROC curve over the entire range of from 0 to 1. When interest is focused on a region of values of the False Positive Rates, the integral is taken only over the particular range and defines the value of the pAUC. For example, if only high values (e.g. 0.8 to 1.0) of specificity are of practical interest, the pAUC is derived by the integral

$$pAUC[0, 0.2] = \int_0^{0.2} ROC(t)dt.$$

It can be shown that for continuous markers (that is, in the theoretical absence of ties), the AUC is also given by,

$$AUC = P(X_1 < X_2). \tag{2.8}$$

As a consequence, the AUC is the probability that, given two measurements, one from the group of non-diseased subjects and one from the group of diseased subjects, the measurement of the non-diseased subject will be smaller than the measurement of the diseased subject.

The AUC and pAUC can be interpreted as average values of test sensitivity estimated over the corresponding range of specificity values. Theoretically, the AUC ranges between 0 and 1. However, if the AUC is below 0.5, the decisions based on the test values can be reversed and result in a new marker with AUC above 0.5. Thus, we will only consider AUC values on the range of 0.5 to 1. AUC values above 0.5 are considered useful in practice, although the level varies across settings. For example, mature diagnostic imaging tests or biomarkers would have AUC above 0.75 in many clinical settings, while many markers may not reach that level, especially in the early development phase (see e.g. Hilden (1991) [121]). For the illustration of Figure 2.3, the AUC for scenario (a) is very close to 0.5, for scenario (b) it is 0.85, while for scenario (c) it is close to one.

An empirical estimate of the AUC can be obtained by using the empirical ROC curve, which, as noted earlier, is obtained by connecting the points $(1-\hat{Spec}(c), \hat{Sens}(c))$ pairs. The resulting AUC estimate is equivalent to (and thus can be estimated by) the Mann-Whitney statistic,

$$\hat{AUC} = \frac{1}{n_1 n_2} \sum_{j=1}^{n_1} \sum_{i=1}^{n_2} I(X_{2i} > X_{1j}), \tag{2.9}$$

where $I(X_{2i} > X_{1j})$ equals one if measurement i from a diseased subject is larger than measurement j from a healthy subject, for all i, j, with $i = 1, \ldots, n_2$ and $j = 1, \ldots, n_1$. When ties between measurements exist, Equation (2.9) becomes:

$$\hat{AUC} = \frac{1}{n_1 n_2} \sum_{j=1}^{n_1} \sum_{i=1}^{n_2} [I(X_{2i} > X_{1j}) + \frac{1}{2} I(X_{2i} = X_{1j})]. \tag{2.10}$$

For the simple example presented in Section 2.2.2.1, the $\hat{AUC}$ is equal to 0.833 since it is the sum of two square areas equal to $(0.5 \times 0.667 + 0.5 \times 1.0)$. Equivalently, using Equation (2.9), the first healthy subject's measurement, 5, is less than all three diseased subjects' measurements $(6, 8, 9)$, while the second healthy subject's measurement, 7, is less than 8 and 9 only. As a result, $\sum_{j=1}^{n_1} \sum_{i=1}^{n_2} I(X_{2i} > X_{1j}) = 3 + 2 = 5$, and $\hat{AUC} = \frac{5}{6}$. Similarly, for the example of Section 2.2.2.2, $\hat{AUC} = 0.93$.

2.2.3.2 Maximum of the Youden index

The value of sensitivity corresponding to a particular value of specificity (or conversely) is of practical interest when it is possible to fix one or the other characteristic by selecting the appropriate threshold for a marker value. When the threshold can be manipulated easily, the value of the *pair* of sensitivity and specificity is a summary of interest.

However, because of the tradeoff between sensitivity and specificity, the question of primary interest is the selection of a threshold on the marker on the basis of an optimality criterion. The maximum of the Youden index is a commonly used criterion and is defined as

$$J = max_c\{Sens(c) + Spec(c) - 1\} = max_c|F_1(c) - F_2(c)|.$$

As noted above, the criterion would select points on the curve which maximize the distance from the curve to the main diagonal, where $Sens = 1 - Spec$.

The empirical estimator of the maximum of the Youden index is defined as

$$J = max_c\{\hat{Sens}(c) + \hat{Spec}(c) - 1\} = max_c|\hat{F}_1(c) - \hat{F}_2(c)| \tag{2.11}$$

and it is equivalent to the Kolmogorov–Smirnov statistic [252]. Inference for the ROC curve based on the empirical estimator of the maximum of the Youden index follows from this equivalence. The procedure is described in detail in Gail, Green (1976) [90]. In practice, the empirical estimator of the maximum of the Youden index is estimated via the computational exercise of calculating

$$\{\hat{Sens}(c) + \hat{Spec}(c) - 1\}$$

for each possible cut-off, c, and picking the maximum of these, or in formal notation: $\arg\max_c\{\hat{Sens}(c) + \hat{Spec}(c) - 1\}$.

The relative importance of sensitivity and specificity for any given problem can be reflected in the choice of the optimal cut-off point by introducing weights, ν and μ, in the general definition of the maximum of the Youden index as follows: $J^* = max_c\{\nu \cdot Sens(c) + \mu \cdot Spec(c) - 1\}$. These weights can be difficult to set in practice [98]. The use of the Youden index has been discussed in a number of articles (e.g. Fluss et al. (2005) [87]; Schisterman and Perkins (2007) [235]; Skaltsa et al. (2010) [245]). Zou et al. (2013) [318] also discuss other possible metrics for obtaining an optimal cut-off point.

Other approaches for the selection of the optimal cut-off point of an ROC curve have also been proposed in the literature. Specifically, the use of a general loss-function was considered by Skaltsa et al. (2010) [245], while Liu (2012) [155] proposed the use of the maximum of the product of sensitivity and specificity. Perkins and Schisterman (2006) [208] compared the Youden index approach with the point-closest-to-(0,1) approach and concluded that the Youden index approach is preferable. The point-closest-to-(0,1) approach for the selection of the optimal ROC-based cut-off point is the point of the ROC curve that corresponds to the minimum Euclidean distance from the ROC curve to the upper left corner of the ROC space, i.e. the point $(1 - Spec(c), Sens(c)) = (0, 1)$. The Youden index approach is undoubtedly the most widely used in practice, and its properties are well-established in the literature.

2.2.3.3 Length of the ROC curve

Another overall accuracy measure discussed in the literature is the length of the ROC curve [20, 89, 184]. Franco-Pereira et al. (2020) [89] discuss the derivation of ROC length in a parametric setting, while Bantis et al. (2021) [20] motivate the concept under a high-throughput data framework aiming to detect markers corresponding to *improper* ROC curves.

ROC curves that are non-concave are defined as "improper." The topic has received attention especially in diagnostic radiology settings (see e.g. [12]). Non-concave ROC curves correspond to cases where the usual monotone ordering $F_1(X) < F_2(X)$ does not consistently hold over the support of marker measurements. This will imply that the ROC curve will cross the main diagonal.

During the early stage of biomarker discovery, a large number of biomarkers might be available. Common measures, such as the AUC and the Youden index, may be suboptimal for detecting markers that. However, the length of the ROC curve is a measure that can overcome the issue of "improperness."

The length of the ROC curve is defined by:

$$l_{ROC} = \int_0^1 \sqrt{1 + \left(\frac{dROC(t)}{dt}\right)^2} dt = \int_{-\infty}^{+\infty} \sqrt{\left(\frac{dFPR(c)}{dc}\right)^2 + \left(\frac{dTPR(c)}{dc}\right)^2} dc \tag{2.12}$$

where $FPR = S_1(c) = 1 - F_1(c)$ and $TPR = S_2(c) = 1 - F_2(c)$ for a given cut-off c. It can also be shown that:

$$l_{ROC} = \int_{-\infty}^{+\infty} \sqrt{1 + \left(\frac{f_2(x)}{f_1(x)}\right)^2} f_1(x)dx = \int_{-\infty}^{+\infty} \sqrt{f_2^2(x) + f_1^2(x)}dx.$$

Here f_1 and f_2 are the probability density functions corresponding to F_1 and F_2, respectively. It can be shown that $\sqrt{2} \leq l_{ROC} < 2$. The minimum value, $\sqrt{2}$, is attained if and only if the distribution of the diseased is identical to that of the non-diseased, which implies a non-informative marker. The quantity $l_{ROC} - \sqrt{2}$, i.e. the difference between the length of the ROC curve and the length of a non-informative marker, is a ϕ-divergence measure, that is, a measure of difference between two probability distributions [20]. Inference under a broad parametric framework and derivation of the asymptotic distribution of the length under the null and alternative hypotheses are discussed in Bantis et al. (2021) [20] and are based on $\phi-$divergence theory (see e.g. [231]). Kernel-based estimators and randomization tests are also discussed in Bantis et al. (2021) [20].

ROC curve essentials

- The ROC curve is the plot that depicts sensitivity vs. 1-specificity for all possible cut-off points c.
- $ROC(c) = (1 - Spec(c), Sens(c)) = (1 - F_1(c), 1 - F_2(c)), c \in (-\infty, \infty)$.
- In functional form, $ROC(t) = 1 - F_2(F_1^{-1}(1 - t)), t \in [0, 1]$.
- AUC is the most widely used metric of overall diagnostic performance of a marker.
- $AUC = P(X_1 < X_2)$.
- Based on elementary calculus, $AUC = \int_0^1 ROC(t)dt$.
- $\hat{AUC} = \frac{1}{n_1 n_2} \sum_{j=1}^{n_1} \sum_{i=1}^{n_2} [I(X_{2i} > X_{1j}) + \frac{1}{2} I(X_{2i} = X_{1j})]$.
- The maximum of the Youden index, $J = max_c\{Sens(c) + Spec(c) - 1\}$, is the largest distance from the ROC curve to the main diagonal.
- The length of the ROC curve is equivalent to a ϕ-divergence measure.

2.3 Graphs and Metrics Related to the ROC Curve

As discussed in this chapter, the ROC curve summarizes all potential pairs of test sensitivity and 1-specificity as the threshold for test positivity ranges across all possible values. Similarly to sensitivity and specificity, the ROC curve is defined and estimated *conditionally* on a binary reference standard and is intended to summarize the diagnostic performance of test.

A variety of extensions of this basic model have been proposed over the years in order (a) to assess diagnostic performance in different settings, (b) to assess predictive performance, or (c) to provide a joint assessment of diagnostic and predictive performance.

The first class of extensions includes methods for assessing the performance of tests in both detection and localization of an abnormality, such as *Free Response ROC Analysis* which will be discussed later on in this section, and methods for assessing diagnostic performance when the reference standard is continuous or discrete taking more than two values. In particular, *ROC surface* methodology addresses diagnosis/classification with a k-class reference standard ($k \geq 3$) as discussed in Chapter 5. The second class of extensions includes methods for assessing the predictive performance of tests, such as *time-dependent ROC analysis* and *predictive ROC curve analysis.* We discuss time-dependent ROC analysis in Chapter 6 of the book and offer a brief description of predictive curve analysis in Sections 2.3.3 and 2.3.4. The third class of extensions is discussed last in this section.

2.3.1 Free-Response ROC analysis (FROC)

The usual ROC model assumes a single test result per case and a binary reference standard about the presence or absence of an abnormality. As such, the model does not consider the issue of correctly localizing a lesion in a scan and does not accommodate the detection of multiple lesions in a single image. Although correct localization considerations can be accommodated within the usual ROC framework by the use of matching by location and segment-level analysis, a more general and methodologically satisfying approach has been developed and proposed under the name of *free-response ROC analysis (FROC).* The FROC model addresses both the detection and localization of multiple lesions from the same participant evaluations [13, 50].

Briefly, in an FROC study, the reader or AI software places marks in locations suspected to contain an abnormality and also generates a degree of suspicion about each mark. If reference standard information is available, as in ROC studies, the presence or absence of a true abnormality is assessed for each of the marked locations. Thus, each marked location would represent a true or a false positive, using a threshold on the distance from the marked location to an actual abnormality as recorded by the reference standard. This threshold is called the *acceptance radius* and is set during the design of the experiment. Also, for a given threshold on the degree of suspicion scale, the test result can be classified as positive or negative. The FROC curve is then defined as the collection of points for which the x-axis coordinate is the average number of false positive points per case, and the y-axis coordinate is the corresponding fraction of correctly detected and localized abnormalities. The reader may consult Bandos et al. (2009) [13] for a discussion of estimation of the area under the FROC curve and Bandos and Obuchowski (2019) [11] for a discussion of how FROC data can be analyzed using ROC methods.

2.3.2 gROC curve

Under the usual setting where the stochastic ordering $F_1(x) < F_2(x)$ holds for all x in the support of both distributions for the densities F_1 and F_2 of non-diseased and diseased subjects, respectively, it is assumed that the higher the measurement, the more likely the existence of disease. In some settings, however, we are interested in capturing markers for which very high and very low measurements are indicative of disease, while measurements of the non-diseased are considered to lie in a possibly bounded interval, say (c_1, c_2). In such cases, an analog to an ROC curve, namely, the generalized ROC (gROC), can be considered and involves redefining the sensitivity, the specificity, and the false positive rates as follows:

$$Sens(c_1, c_2) = F_2(c_1) + S_2(c_2),$$
$$Spec(c_1, c_2) = F_1(c_2) - F_1(c_1),$$
$$FPR(c_1, c_2) = F_1(c_1) + S_1(c_2),$$

where $c_1 < c_2$. To perform an ROC analysis, one can plot two surfaces in the unit cube, one that refers to the sensitivity and one that refers to the specificity for all $c_1 < c_2$, $c_i \in (-\infty, +\infty)$, $i = 1, 2$. Bantis et al. (2021) [20] illustrate these plots with real data examples.

The *generalized* ROC curve (gROC) is defined as [163, 164]:

$$\begin{aligned} gROC(t) &= \sup_{F_1(c_1)+S_1(c_2)=t} \{F_2(c_1) + S_2(c_2)\} = \sup_{c_1 \leq F_1^{-1}(t)} \{Sens(t; c_1)\} \\ &= \sup_{c_1 \leq F_1^{-1}(t)} \{F_2(c_1) + ROC\,(t - F_1(c_1))\} \quad t \in (0, 1). \end{aligned} \tag{2.13}$$

In addition, the respective gROC Youden index can be defined that allows for optimal cut-off point derivation [20]:

$$gJ = max_{c_1, c_2} \{Se(c_1, c_2) + Sp(c_1, c_2) - 1\}$$

It is of note that, under the condition of a unimodal density ratio, the gROC is optimal, in the sense of achieving a maximum AUC, and its length is the same with the corresponding standard ROC curve [20] (see Figure 2.4).

2.3.3 Net benefit approaches and decision curve analysis

Prediction models, diagnostic tests, and molecular markers are traditionally evaluated using statistics such as sensitivity and specificity. Decision analysis goes one step further and attempts to assess clinical value by incorporating clinical consequences, such as the benefit of finding disease early or the harm of unnecessary further testing. Net benefit is a simple type of decision analysis which can be plotted against a range of exchange rates in what is called a "decision curve" [253]. Decision curves are used in the literature to evaluate whether clinical use of prediction models, diagnostic tests, and molecular markers would do more good than harm. The concept was introduced in the article of Vickers and Elkin (2006) [276] and is further described in Vickers et al. (2016, 2019) [277, 278] among others. Code and a manual for implementation in `R` and `Stata` can be found in `https://www.mskcc.org/departments/epidemiology-biostatistics/biostatistics/decision-curve-analysis`.

2.3.4 Predictive ROC (PROC) curve

As discussed earlier in this chapter, the ROC curve is defined and estimated conditionally on the true disease status, as are the sensitivity and the

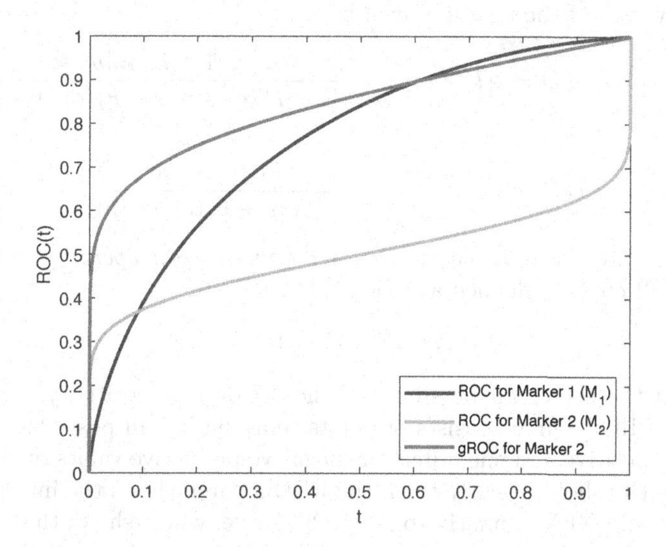

FIGURE 2.4
An illustration of ROC and gROC curves for hypothetical markers M_1 and M_2. M_1 visually appears to outperform M_2 in terms of AUC. The gROC of M_2, however, results in an AUC higher that the one of the ROC of M_1. The gROC of M_2 and the ROC of M_2 have exactly the same length.

specificity of the test or marker. As such, these three measures of diagnostic performance are considered to be invariant to disease prevalence and, theoretically, could be transported from one prevalence setting to another. By contrast, measures of the predictive value of a marker, such at the positive and negative predictive values are defined conditionally on the test result and as a simple calculation shows, they vary across cohorts with different disease prevalence. This fundamental distinction between diagnosis (detection) and prediction is an essential aspect of the evaluation of a marker and affects the design, analysis, and interpretation of studies.

The result of a test or marker becomes binary typically after the application of a threshold for declaring test positivity. The assessment of the possible pairs of sensitivity and 1-specificity across all possible threshold gives rise to the ROC curve. In this section we discuss the prediction analog of the ROC curve, which characterizes the set of positive and negative predictive values of the test as the threshold for test positivity varies, which was introduced by Shiu and Gatsonis (2008) [242].

If D represents binary disease status (1=non-diseased, 2=diseased) and T the test result, let F_2 and F_1 denote the cumulative density functions of $T|D = 2$ and $T|D = 1$, respectively. Note that the disease prevalence is $p = Pr(D = 2)$. For a test positivity threshold c, the positive and negative predictive values of the test are given by

$$PPV(c) = Pr(D = 2|T \geq c) = \frac{[1 - F_2(c)]p}{[1 - F_2(c)]p + [1 - F_1(c)](1 - p)}, \tag{2.14}$$

$$NPV(c) = Pr(D = 1|T < c) = \frac{F_1(c)(1 - p)}{F_2(c)p + F_1(c)(1 - p)}. \tag{2.15}$$

In analogy to the ROC curve, the *predictive receiver operating characteristic* (PROC) curve is defined as follows:

$$\{(1 - NPV(c), PPV(c))\}_{c \in R},$$

where R is the set of all possible thresholds for test positivity. Thus, the theoretical PROC curve consists of points representing all possible combinations of the positive and one minus the negative predictive values obtained by varying the threshold. Clearly then, the PROC curve shows the interplay between PPV and NPV similarly to the ROC curve, which shows the interplay between test sensitivity and specificity. The collection of observed (1-NPV, PPV) points defines the *empirical* PROC curve.

The geometry of PROC curves is surprisingly complex. For example, these curves may not be monotonic, that is may not display a one-to-one correspondence between PPV and NPV, even for many parameter configurations in the binormal setting. Thus, two different PPV values may be feasible for the same NPV value. Shiu and Gatsonis (2008) [242] provide conditions for the monotonicity of the PROC curve and discuss the estimation of the curve using pseudolikelihood methods. The geometric complexity of the PROC curve reflects the fact that the interplay between PPV and NPV of a test is also complex. As a corollary, the use of PPV and NPV curves *separately*, as proposed for example in Moskowitz and Pepe (2004) [179], can be misleading because it does not take into account the pattern of the two quantities as the threshold varies and, may consider pairs of values of the two quantities that *are not feasible.*

2.3.5 Precision-Recall curve

The third class of extensions includes methods intended to assess the combined diagnostic and predictive performance of a test. An often-used approach is based on the *Precision-Recall curve.* The PR curve consists of all possible pairs of the positive predictive value (*Recall*, in machine learning terminology), and the sensitivity (*Precision* in machine learning terminology) of a test as the threshold for test positivity varies across all possible values. The PR curve is fundamentally a graphical device depicting the relation of test sensitivity and PPV, without the intrinsic interpretation of the ROC curve and its summaries. For example, whereas the area under the ROC curve has a direct interpretation as the probability of correct ranking of cases with and without the target condition, there is no such interpretation for the PR curve [177].

Precision-Recall curves have been used in areas of machine learning, notably in information retrieval, where empirical studies showed that as recall increases, precision would decrease [44]. The pattern of the relation between PPV and sensitivity is not necessarily monotone and the PR curves can be rather complex, especially near the boundary values of sensitivity and PPV. In addition, a part of the PR space is not achievable by the curve [38]. Parametric and nonparametric methods for estimating the PR curve and its functionals have been developed [37, 137] and can be implemented via available software [97]. In particular, the area under the PR curve has been proposed as a measure of the performance of systems [62, 230].

Because the PR curve combines a diagnostic quantity (sensitivity/precision) with a predictive quantity (PPV/recall), the curve is defined and estimated conditionally on both margins of the traditional 2×2 table for diagnostic tests. Thus direct estimates of the curve can be obtained only from a limited range of study designs. In particular, direct estimates cannot be obtained from the widely used designs in which one of the margins is fixed. This limitation of the PR curve is not simply technical but stems from the limited utility of the curve in the assessment of diagnostic accuracy or predictive accuracy of a modality. As a consequence, the PR curve has not been used extensively in the evaluation of medical tests.

Despite the utility of ROC curves, two issues can arise in the presence of highly imbalanced sample sizes between diseased and non-diseased subjects. The first is that with few diseased subjects recall will increase quickly as diseased subjects are tracked. This can lead to big differences in ROC/AUC for small changes where the positive cases lie in the ranked list. Also, small changes in the False Positive Rate indicate large changes in the number of false positives when there are many more non-diseased subjects in the study. The second issue is that, there can be settings where ROC/AUC is increasing for highly imbalanced sample sizes between diseased and non-diseased subjects [55]. Precision-recall curves incorporate the information of disease prevalence in the assessment of a diagnostic marker. As a result, they can be misleading if directly used with data arising from a designed case–control study given that prevalence is not properly estimated from the data at hand. A separate estimation for PPV is needed first.

Figure 2.5 illustrates a PR curve based on data from the DMIST study, along with the corresponding ROC curve for a selected, specific reader, modality, and machine. The classification variable used is the subjective probability of malignancy as assessed by the specific reader, while the presence of breast cancer is the reference standard. The corresponding `Stata` output from the results window follows. Notice that, the prevalence of disease is estimated from the data at hand. Such an estimate is appropriate when the design of the study allows for this based on the sampling strategy used for data collection.

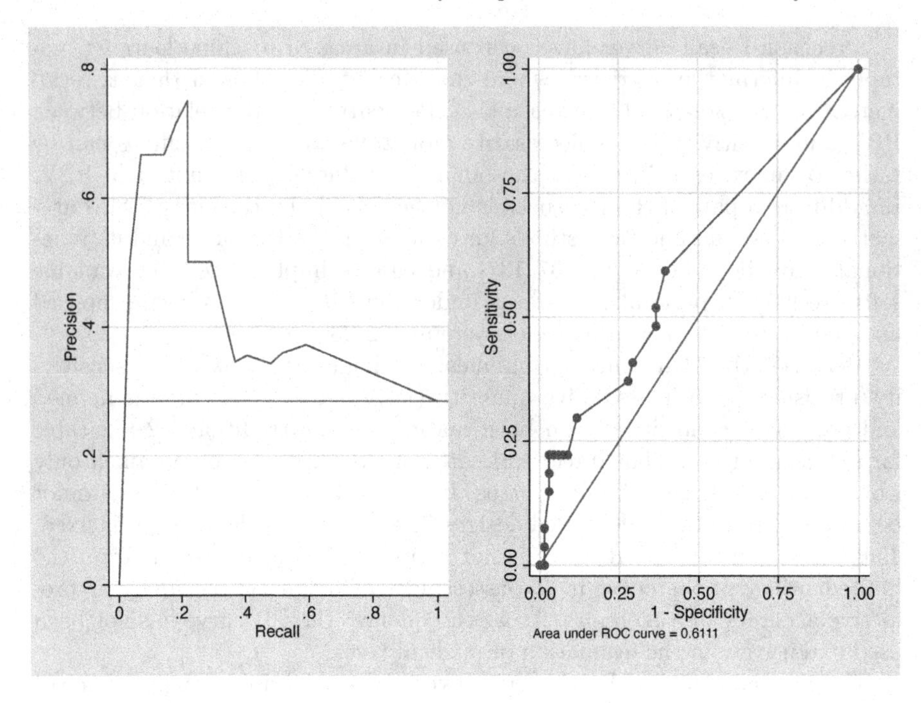

FIGURE 2.5
Precision-recall curve for the DMIST data (left panel) and respective ROC curve (right panel).

```
. net sj 20-1
.  net install st0591

. prcurve cancer pmalig if readerid==2 & modality==2 & machine==2

         Number of observations        =  95
         Unique values of classifier   =  17
         Number of positive cases      =  27
         Portion of positive cases     =  0.2842

--------------------------------------------------
   Recall =  0.1481     0.2222     0.3704
--------------------------------------------------
 Precision   0.6667     0.7500     0.3448
--------------------------------------------------

 Area under precision-recall curve:  0.4246

 . roctab cancer pmalig if readerid==2 & modality==2 & machine==2, graph
```

2.4 Illustrations

In this section, we provide some illustative numerical examples using `R` and `Stata`. An `R` package offering a variety of useful tools for visualizing, assessing, and interpreting ROC curves is `pROC` [221], while `ROCR` [244] is dedicated to ROC curve analysis from the machine learning perspective. The latter package supports the calculation of the measures of Table 2.2 and also provides the corresponding standard evaluation plots, such as ROC curves that will be the main topic of this book and Precision/Recall plots that depict the tradeoff between Recall (sensitivity) and Precision (PPV).

2.4.1 Continuous-scaled marker

We use part of the CD4 marker dataset (Brucellosis study, Section 1.4.1) in order to illustrate the construction of diagnostic and predictive performance measures and the ROC curve for a continuous-scaled marker.

CD4 measurements for the 15 Controls were

$$\{59, 66, 45, 62, 51, 50, 49, 58, 53, 42, 50, 47, 51, 62, 48\}$$

while respective measurements for the 12 Acute Brucellosis Cases were

$$\{72, 70, 69, 82, 68, 59, 76, 61, 59, 73, 49, 77\}.$$

Suppose that we choose $c = 61$, thus considering measurements larger than or equal to 61 as diseased and measurements smaller than 61 as healthy. Then, the sensitivity is equal to 75% (i.e. 9/12), while the specificity is 80% (i.e. 12/15). Also, $LR(+) = 3.75$ and $LR(-) = 0.31$.

Observed values of sensitivity and specificity and the empirical ROC curve are shown in Figure 2.6.

Note: The figure shows the ROC curve in the usual coordinates of ROC space and also with specificity in the x-axis instead of 1-specificity. The latter presentation may be occasionally useful.

The ROC curve can be generated through the `'Graphics --> ROC Analysis'` menu in Stata or via the `roctab` command from the Stata Command line: `roctab` <*Reference variable*> <*Classification variable*>, `graph summary`.

The output also offers a 95% confidence interval for the AUC. Specifically, $P(0.752 < AUC < 1.000) = 0.95$. Based on this result for AUC, we conclude that CD4 is a useful diagnostic marker for the diagnosis of acute brucellosis relative to controls.

Implementation in `R` using the `pROC` or the `ROCR` packages provides similar results. Figure 2.8 displays the graphical output using either `pROC` or `ROCR`. By default, `pROC` plots specificity instead of 1-specificity on the x-axis but with the axis reversed. This choice may be considered to be a neat way to

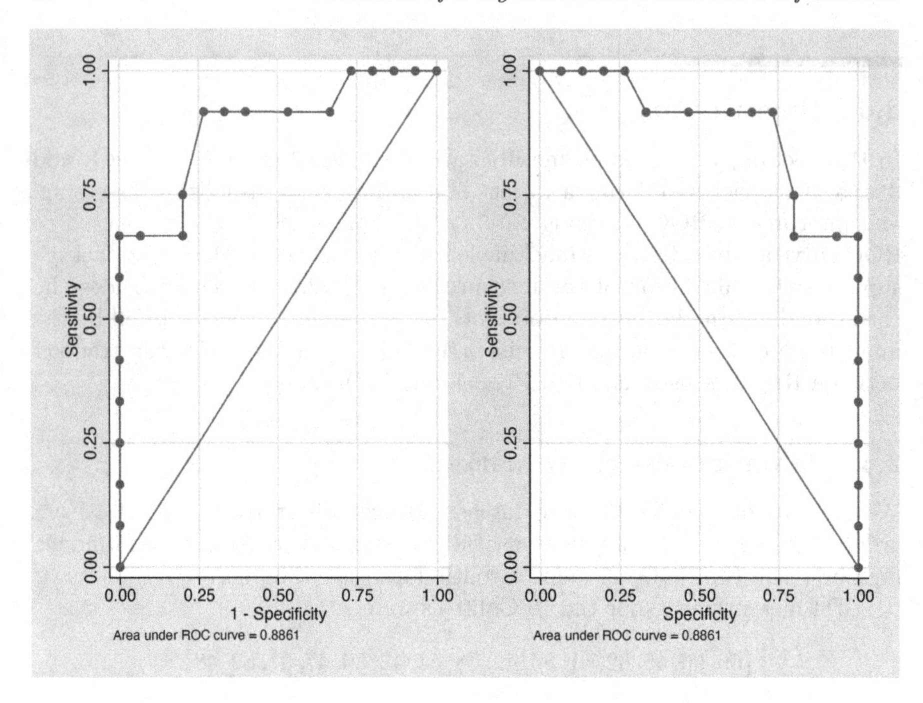

FIGURE 2.6
ROC curve for marker CD4 peripheral blood count (left panel) and respective sens vs spec graph (right panel).

capture the trade-off between sensitivity and specificity but may also seem a bit awkward because of the reversed axis. Of course, there is an option to plot the ROC curve in the conventional way (using the `legacy.axes=TRUE` argument in the relevant `plot.roc` function). `ROCR` offers the option to depict a color gradient on the ROC curve according to the biomarker measurements which are given as a second y-axis on the right-hand side of the graph. `R` code for the implementation along with respective output follow.

```
library(pROC)

brucd4con<-c(59, 66, 45, 62, 51, 50, 49, 58, 53, 42, 50, 47,
51, 62, 48)
brucd4cas<-c(72, 70, 69, 82, 68, 59, 76, 61, 59, 73, 49, 77)

roc(controls=brucd4con,cases=brucd4cas, plot=T, ci=T)

library(ROCR)

pred <- prediction(c(brucd4con,brucd4cas), c(rep(0,15),rep(1,12)))
```

```
perf <- performance(pred,"tpr","fpr")

plot(perf,colorize=TRUE)

areaest<-performance(pred,"auc")
areaest@y.values    #provides AUC
```

```
## Setting direction: controls < cases

## Call:
## roc.default(controls = brucd4con, cases = brucd4cas, ci = T, plot = T)

## Data: 15 controls < 12 cases.
## Area under the curve: 0.8861
## 95% CI: 0.7523-1 (DeLong)


## > areaest@y.values
## [[1]]
## [1] 0.8861111
```

Although the calculation of estimates of PPV and NPV is straightforward using the available data, the population interpretation of the estimates needs

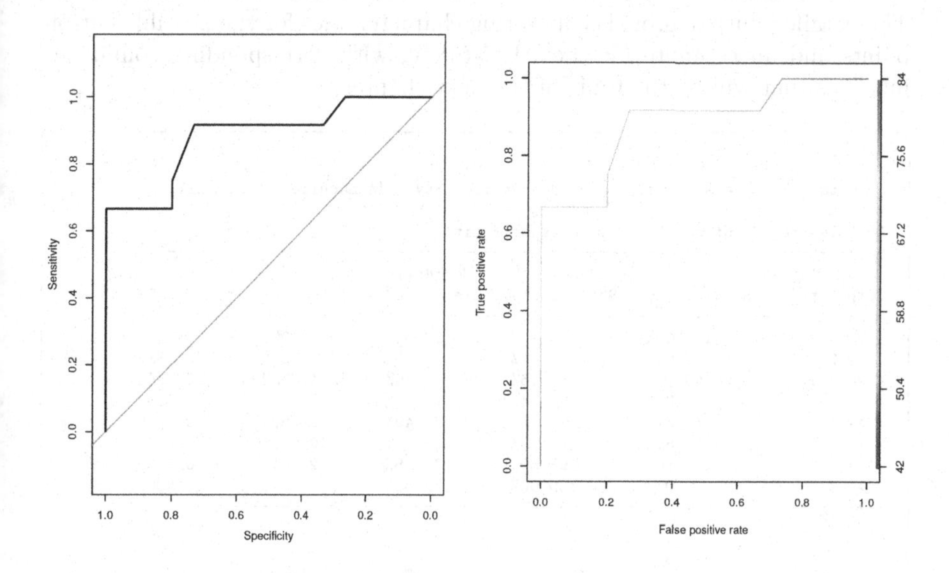

FIGURE 2.7
ROC curve for CD4 using `pROC` (left panel) and `ROCR` (right panel) `R`-packages.

to consider that the estimates are derived from a population with the observed prevalence of disease. Suppose that the prevalence of disease in the target population is 2%. Then, $PPV = 7.11\%$, while $NPV = 99.37\%$. Predictive values are calculated based on the assumption that the prior probability of a positive test result based on the reference standard is just 2%, equal to the prevalence of disease. Correct estimation of the prevalence in the target population is crucial for the correct estimation of PPV, NPV in turn. For example, if the prevalence is actually 5%, then $PPV = 16.48\%$, while $NPV = 98.38\%$. (PPV, NPV can be calculated using the Bayes formula on a spreadsheet).

Estimates of prevalence are not possible in designed case–control studies (as in the Brucellosis example). In cohort studies, where a cohort from the population of interest is followed and population characteristics and disease status are recorded, the estimation is straightforward (as number of diseased over number of subjects in the study). Valid estimates of prevalence can also be provided through epidemiological studies in the target population.

2.4.2 Ordinal-scaled marker

Data from the DIMST study discussed in Section 1.4.5 are used for this illustration. Data are given in Table 2.7. Higher scores are indicative of disease. The reader assessed images from 98 subjects and gave a score from 1 (less indicative of disease) to 7 (more indicative of disease). The true status of each subject was evaluated with a biopsy.

Necessarily, the resulting ROC curve will be defined by eight possible sensitivity, specificity pairs as shown in the Stata results window that follows. The detailed output provides operating characteristics for the possible cut-off points and an estimate for the AUC (along with corresponding confidence intervals that will be the topic of the next chapter).

```
. roctab cancer ptscore if readerid ==2& modality ==1& machine ==2, detail

Detailed report of sensitivity and specificity
------------------------------------------------------------------------------
                                          Correctly
Cutpoint      Sensitivity   Specificity   Classified          LR+          LR-
------------------------------------------------------------------------------
( >= 1 )          100.00%         0.00%       27.55%       1.0000
( >= 2 )           51.85%        70.42%       65.31%       1.7531       0.6837
( >= 3 )           48.15%        74.65%       67.35%       1.8992       0.6946
( >= 4 )           37.04%        90.14%       75.51%       3.7566       0.6985
( >= 5 )           14.81%        97.18%       74.49%       5.2593       0.8765
( >= 6 )           14.81%        98.59%       75.51%      10.5185       0.8640
( >= 7 )            3.70%        98.59%       72.45%       2.6296       0.9767
( >  7 )            0.00%       100.00%       72.45%                    1.0000
------------------------------------------------------------------------------


                      ROC                    -Asymptotic Normal--
           Obs       Area     Std. Err.      [95% Conf. Interval]
     ------------------------------------------------------------
```

TABLE 2.7
Contingency table for the assessment of screen-film imaging for breast cancer by true disease state from the DMIST study. Numbers represent frequencies.

True disease status *vs.* score	1	2	3	4	5	6	7
D_1	50	3	11	5	1	0	1
D_2	13	1	3	6	0	3	1

```
          98       0.6424          0.0605          0.52385      0.76097

. roctab cancer ptscore if readerid==2 & modality==1 & machine==2, graph
```

2.4.3 Binary-scaled marker

Evaluation of an antigen-based rapid test for the diagnosis of SARS-CoV-2 presence in respiratory samples was performed in Porte et al (2020) [214]. A

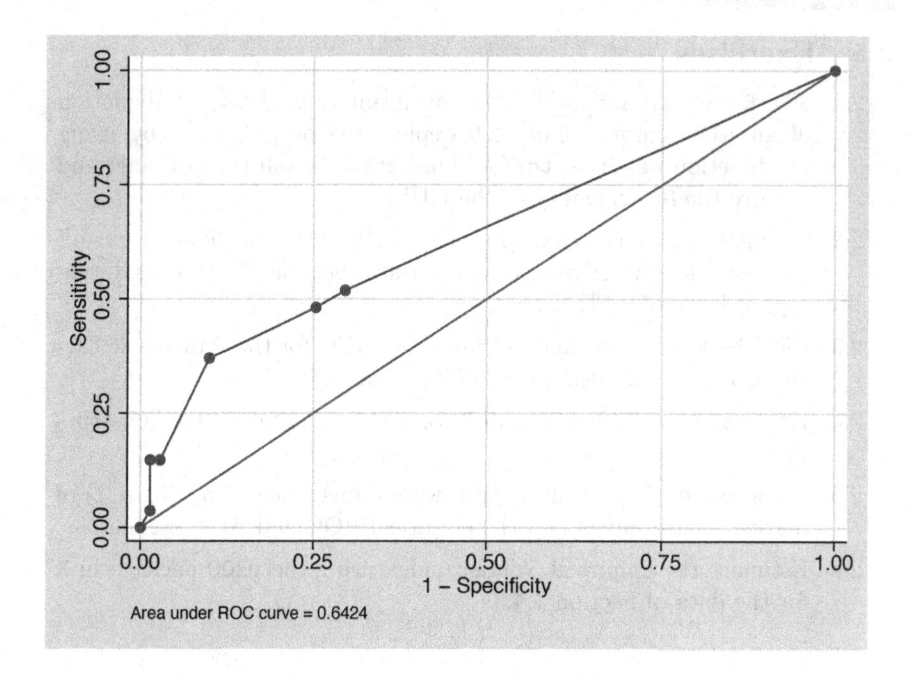

FIGURE 2.8
ROC curve for screen-film imaging for breast cancer. For an ordinal-scaled marker, for a k point scale there are $k+1$ possible cut-offs.

TABLE 2.8
Contingency table for a binary diagnostic marker. Numbers represent frequencies.

	Negative test: T_1	Positive test: T_2
D_1	45	0
D_2	5	77

total of 127 subjects were tested. The reference standard was RT-PCR, which resulted in 45 negative and 82 positive results, while the antigen detection test resulted in 50 negative and 77 positive results. The corresponding contingency table is given in Table 2.8.

As a result, test sensitivity is estimated to be equal to 93.9% (95% CI: 86.5%, 97.4%), with corresponding specificity equal to 100%. Confidence intervals for sensitivity were calculated in `Stata` using the `prtesti` command. For an estimate of prevalence equal to 9%, estimated PPV, NPV are equal to 100% and 99.4%, respectively.

2.5 Exercises

2.1 The `R` package `asbio` [2] offers an intuitive GUI for the depiction of an ROC curve. Figure 2.9 depicts the output given by using the function `see.roc.tck()` from `asbio`. Install the package, and explore the functionality of the GUI.

2.2 Calculate the sensitivity, specificity, PPV, NPV for different cut-off points of the Pancreatic carcinoma data (Section 1.4.3), considering a prevalence of 0.5%.

2.3 Plot the ROC curve and calculate the AUC for the Pancreatic carcinoma data (e.g. using the `ROCR` package).

2.4 Explore the `pROC` package in `R` for empirical ROC curve construction.

2.5 Explore the effect of linear transformations (such as $y = 5x + 7$) of marker measurements on the empirical ROC and AUC estimates.

2.6 Estimate the empirical Youden index using the `pROC` package in `R` for the data of Section 1.4.3.

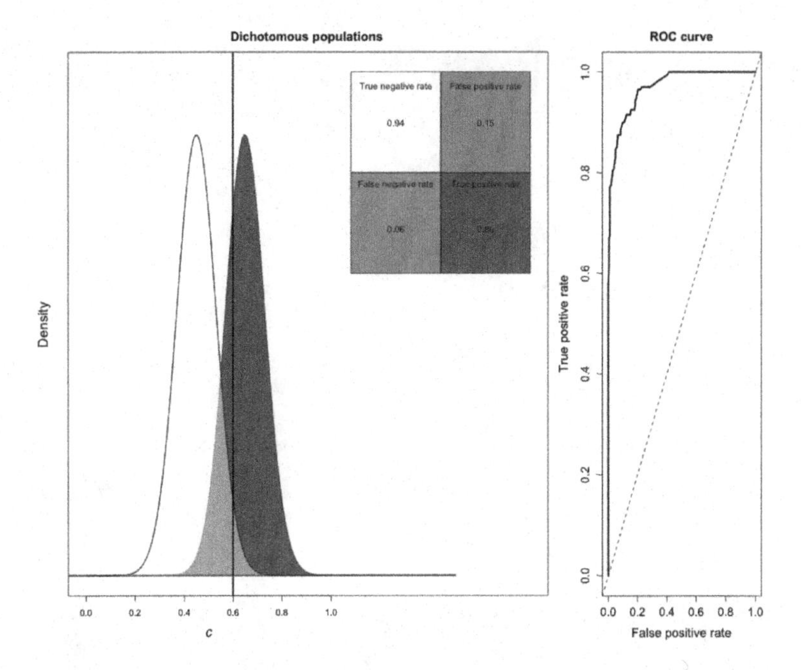

FIGURE 2.9
ROC curve illustration using the `asbio` package in `R`. Several measurements from each distribution depicted on the left panel are drawn and the corresponding empirical ROC curve is constructed on the right panel.

3

Statistical Inference for the ROC Curve

CONTENTS

3.1 Statistical Models for the ROC Curve 48
3.1.1 Binormal and other parametric models 48
3.1.1.1 The Box-Cox transformation in the ROC curve context 51
3.1.1.2 ROC curve estimation for the binormal model via ordinal regression: ordinal marker measurements 54
3.1.1.3 ROC estimation for continuous-scaled data without distributional assumptions 57
3.1.1.4 Pointwise confidence bands for ROC curves derived from continuous marker data 58
3.1.2 Inference for the empirical ROC curve 60
3.1.2.1 Hypothesis testing for the empirical ROC curve 62
3.1.3 Nonparametric models 63
3.1.3.1 Kernel-based ROCs 63
3.1.3.2 Spline-based ROCs 66
3.2 Inference for ROC Summary Measures 70
3.2.1 Statistical inference for the AUC 71
3.2.1.1 Nonparametric methods 71
3.2.1.2 Parametric methods 72
3.2.1.3 Bootstrap-based inference for AUC 74
3.2.2 Hypothesis testing for AUC 75
3.2.3 Statistical inference for the partial Area Under the ROC Curve (pAUC) 77
3.2.4 Selection of optimal points and cut-offs, Youden index . 78
3.2.5 Sensitivity and Specificity at specific cut-off points 81
3.3 Exercises 83

DOI: 10.1201/9780429170140-3

3.1 Statistical Models for the ROC Curve

3.1.1 Binormal and other parametric models

The *binormal* model played an important role in the early formulation and development of ROC analysis [68, 69]. The model is simplest to describe when marker values can be treated as continuous variables. In particular marker values from n_1 non-diseased and n_2 diseased subjects are assumed to follow normal distributions $X_1 \sim N(\mu_1, \sigma_1^2)$ and $X_2 \sim N(\mu_2, \sigma_2^2)$, respectively. By convention we will assume that "diseased" status is associated with larger expected values of the marker, and therefore $\mu_1 \leq \mu_2$. The separation between the two densities provides a measure of the ability of the marker to distinguish and, thus, classify correctly individuals into one of the two groups.

The ROC curve actually depends on the four parameters of the binormal model only through the standardized difference of the means $a = \frac{\mu_2 - \mu_1}{\sigma_2}$, and the ratio of the standard deviations $b = \frac{\sigma_1}{\sigma_2}$. Using the parameters a and b, the curve is defined as

$$ROC(t) = \Phi(a + b\Phi^{-1}(t)), t \in [0, 1]. \tag{3.1}$$

This form of the curve is obtained by applying the general Equation (2.6) discussed on Chapter 2. The reader can verify that, for each cut-off point c, the sensitivity of the marker is given by the equation $sens(c) = \Phi(\frac{\mu_2 - c}{\sigma_2})$ and the specificity by the equation $spec(c) = \Phi(\frac{c - \mu_1}{\sigma_1})$.

The parameter a is often called the *intercept* of the curve, and the parameter b is called the *slope* of the curve. This nomenclature derives from the fact that if the two axes in the ROC plot were transformed via the inverse normal distribution function, the ROC curve would be a straight line with intercept a and slope b [255]. We will return to this terminology in the discussion of fitting ROC curves via ordinal regression. The slope of the curve is also called the *shape* parameter. A symmetric ROC curve corresponds to a shape parameter $b = 1$. Deviations from the value 1 indicate the degree of asymmetry in the curve, as shown in Figure 3.1. If b is fixed, then large values of the location parameter a indicate more steep rise in the ROC curve. Inference for a and b can be based on asymptotic normality assumptions and the use of

$$\hat{Var}(a) = \frac{1}{n_2} + \frac{a^2}{2n_2} + \frac{b^2}{n_1}, \tag{3.2}$$

$$\hat{Var}(b) = \frac{b^2}{2}(\frac{1}{n_2} + \frac{1}{n_1}). \tag{3.3}$$

The latter formulas for the estimation of the variances of a and b can be derived by applying the delta method as in Noll et al. (2019) [193].

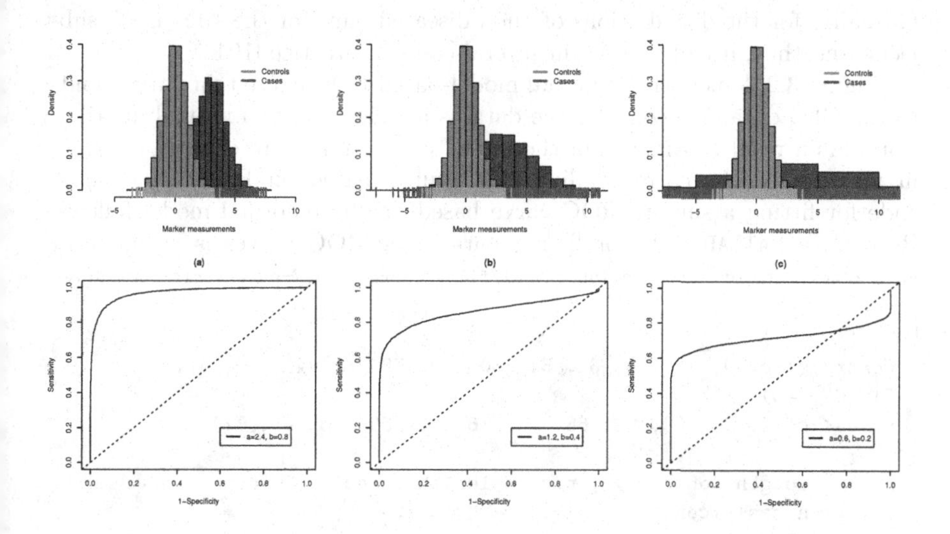

FIGURE 3.1
Binormal ROC curves according to the parameter values a (intercept) & b (slope). The degree of asymmetry in the curve is driven by the slope parameter b. Mean values for cases and controls are kept constant for panels (a), (b), (c), with $\mu_1 = 0$ and $\mu_2 = 3$ in all cases.

If $\frac{\sigma_1}{\sigma_2} = 1$, then the binormal ROC curve is concave and lies above the main diagonal in the unit square. This is a desirable property for the ROC curve because it implies that diseased subjects consistently have higher measurements than non-diseased subjects, and the trade-off between sensitivity and specificity is monotone throughout the range of the curve. In several occasions in practice, this is a reasonable assumption. However, quite often in practice, the binormal model results in $\frac{\sigma_1}{\sigma_2} \neq 1$. As a consequence, the ROC curve crosses the main diagonal and, strictly speaking, implies that both the sensitivity and the specificity of the marker are increasing for a range of threshold values. As noted in Chapter 2, ROC curves with this property have been called "improper" [34]. A number of authors have presented approaches to overcome the difficulties and develop "proper" ROC curves. A nice discussion and a proposal to consider is the use of the bi-gamma model presented in Dorfman et al. (1997) [72].

Although the assumption specifying that marker values follow normal distributions lends simplicity to the model, in practice it would be rather restrictive if it was required to hold strictly. Indeed, the assumption can be relaxed to require only the existence of a monotone transformation that makes both distributions marginally normal [170,318]. Transformations to normality were also used to assess robustness to departures from normality. The binormal model for the ROC curve has been shown to be robust to departures from normality for the distributions of "non-diseased" and/or the "diseased" subjects, and thus, it can be used in several cases in practice [104].

Figure 3.2 depicts the binormal model-based ROC curve that corresponds to the CD4 data. We consider the data as arising from two normal distributions. As a result, estimates of the model parameters were directly plugged-in to produce the corresponding ROC curve based on Equation (3.1). R code for fitting a smooth ROC curve based on the binormal model follows. Respective MATLAB code for fitting parametric ROC curves is available at http://www.mathworks.com/matlabcentral/fileexchange/39127-parametric-roc-curve.

```
controls<-c(59, 66, 45, 62, 51, 50, 49, 58, 53, 42, 50, 47,
51, 62, 48)
cases<-c(72, 70, 69, 82, 68, 59, 76, 61, 59, 73, 49, 77)

n.con<-length(controls) ; n.cas<-length(cases)
n.tot<-n.cas+n.con

mucon<-mean(controls) ; mucas<-mean(cases)
sdcon<-sd(controls) ; sdcas<-sd(cases)

fpseq<-seq(0,1,0.001)

tpseq<-pnorm((mucas-mucon+sdcon*qnorm(fpseq))/sdcas)

subj<-unique(sort(c(controls,cases)))
subj.con<-unique(sort(controls))
subj.cas<-unique(sort(cases))
n.tot<-length(subj)

tp<-rep(0,n.tot); fp<-rep(0,n.tot)

for (i in 1:n.tot){
  tp[i]<-sum(cases >= subj[i])/n.cas
  fp[i]<-sum(controls >= subj[i])/n.con
}

tp<-c(1,tp,0) ; fp<-c(1,fp,0)

plot(fpseq,tpseq, type='l', xlab="1-Specificity",
ylab="Sensitivity")
par(new=T)
abline(0,1, lty=2)
par(new=T)
plot(fp,tp,xlab="",ylab="")
```

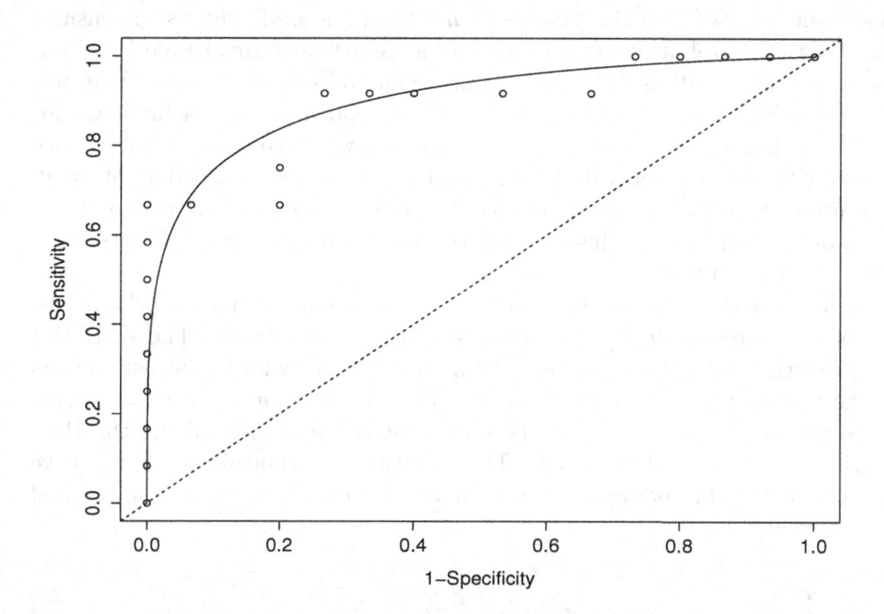

FIGURE 3.2
Binormal model ROC curve for the CD4 data. Points that define the empirical (1-specificity, sensitivity) pairs are also shown for reference.

3.1.1.1 The Box-Cox transformation in the ROC curve context

A systematic way to implement the binormal model utilizes the Box-Cox transformation. The approach was introduced by Zou and Hall (2000) [317] and has been shown to perform well in the ROC context [87, 318].

To derive an appropriate transformation, we consider variables of the form

$$X_1^{(\lambda)} = \begin{cases} \frac{X_1^\lambda - 1}{\lambda}, & \lambda \neq 0 \\ \log(X_1), & \lambda = 0. \end{cases}$$

and similarly for $X_2^{(\lambda)}$. The goal in the ROC curve context is to derive a single value of λ for which both $X_1^{(\lambda)}$ and $X_2^{(\lambda)}$ are independently normally distributed with parameters $\mu_{1(\lambda)}$,$\sigma_{1(\lambda)}$ and $\mu_{2(\lambda)}$, $\sigma_{2(\lambda)}$, respectively.

The common λ can be estimated by maximizing the following profile log-likelihood:

$$l(\lambda) = -\frac{n_1}{2}\log[\frac{\Sigma_{j=1}^{n_1}(X_{1j}^{(\lambda)} - \frac{\Sigma_{j=1}^{n_1} X_{1j}^{(\lambda)}}{n_1})^2}{n_1}] - \frac{n_2}{2}\log[\frac{\Sigma_{i=1}^{n_2}(X_{2i}^{(\lambda)} - \frac{\Sigma_{i=1}^{n_2} X_{2i}^{(\lambda)}}{n_2})^2}{n_2}]$$
$$+(\lambda - 1)(\Sigma_{j=1}^{n_1}\log X_{1j} + \Sigma_{i=1}^{n_2}\log X_{2i}) + k$$

where k is constant.

This specific formulation of the Box-Cox model in the ROC context results in a single value of λ for the "diseased" and "non-diseased" groups and ensures that the two sets of measurements are on the same transformed scale. As a consequence, the resulting ROC curve is invariant to monotone transformations. The Box-Cox transformation as described here, normalizes measurements for both populations of diseased and non-diseased while keeping the invariance property for the empirical ROC that can be constructed by the data at hand. The use of this approach requires modification of standard software but the additional complexity is justified by the fact that the approach corrects a common error in analyses.

R code for the implementation of the Box-Cox transformation prior to the use of the binormal model for continuous data is given below. The sTREM-1 data (Section 1.4.2) are used here. Assuming normality for the measurements of the two groups results in a binormal ROC curve that has a much poorer fit to the empirical ROC than the one constructed after applying the Box-Cox transformation (Figure 3.3). The resulting binormal model ROC curve provides a suitable parametric alternative that closely captures the original data formulation.

```
 trem1x<-c(47.00, 69.54, 72.57, 74.87, 76.42, 76.42, 80.33,
  81.92, 90.80, 94.10, 106.80, 122.70, 123.60, 124.50,
  139.20, 166.10, 180.90, 181.70, 280.90, 307.20, 552.90)
 trem1y<-c(99.12, 178.20, 189.70, 213.90, 248.10, 260.80,
  298.70, 435.30, 67.30, 810.90, 77.20, 104.20, 105.90,
  109.40, 120.00, 124.40, 132.70, 147.50, 151.70, 159.30,
  162.70, 189.70, 191.40, 197.70, 203.90, 275.90, 286.00,
  287.70, 375.40, 488.20)

x<-trem1x ; y<-trem1y
n<-length(x) ; m<-length(y)

roxlik<-function(h)
{
  xh<-((x^h)-1)/h
  yh<-((y^h)-1)/h
loglik<- -(-n/2*log(sum((xh-sum(xh)/n)^2)/n)-
m/2*log(sum((yh-sum(yh)/m)^2)/m)
+(h-1)*(sum(log(x))+sum(log(y))))
return(loglik)
}

parto<- nlm(roxlik,h<-1)
lambda<-parto$estimate

roxcox <- function(x,y,lambda)
 {
```

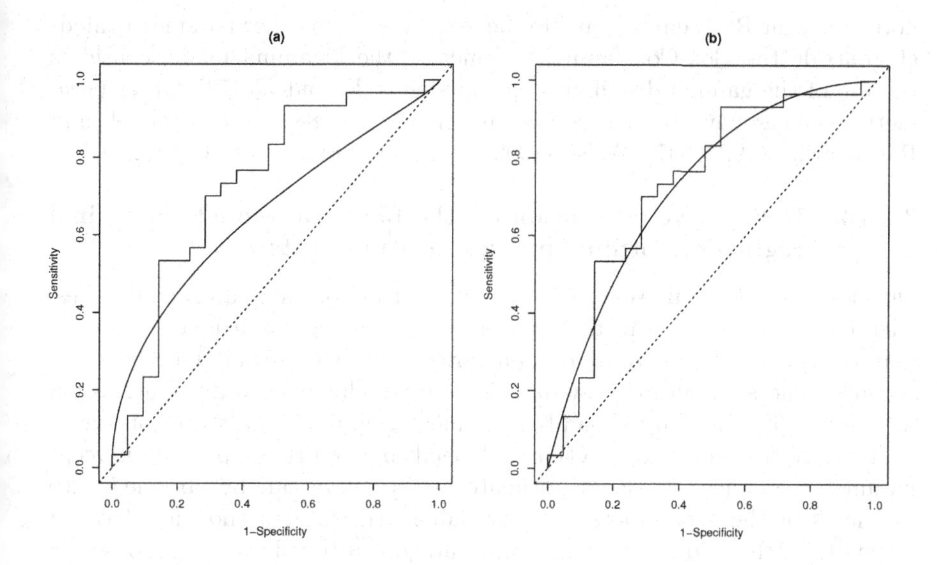

FIGURE 3.3
(a) Smooth ROC cuve based on normality assumptions for marker measurements. (b) Similarly after the ROC curve framework Box-Cox transformation. The corresponding empirical ROC curve is shown for reference.

```
xbc<-((x^lambda)-1)/lambda
ybc<-((y^lambda)-1)/lambda

   return(list(xbc,ybc))
 }

 binormals<-roxcox(x,y,lambda)
```

```
## [[1]]
## [1] 1.875252 1.943465 1.950218 1.955080 1.958237 1.958237 1.965810 1.968740
## [9] 1.983725 1.988769 2.006042 2.023922 2.024835 2.025737 2.039272 2.059407
## [17] 2.068597 2.069063 2.110952 2.118624 2.162252

## [[2]]
## [1] 1.995975 2.067003 2.073567 2.085682 2.099806 2.104359 2.116251 2.145824
## [9] 1.938196 2.185266 1.959791 2.002753 2.004917 2.009218 2.021127 2.025637
## [17] 2.033553 2.046043 2.049265 2.054782 2.057129 2.073567 2.074489 2.077806
## [25] 2.080926 2.109377 2.112519 2.113032 2.134769 2.153915
```

The method discussed above can be used to derive an estimate of the ROC curve for continuous data as transformed by the Box-Cox transformation. We note here that ROC curves can also be estimated from other parametric models, outside the Box-Cox family. Specifically, the bigamma model considers the use of the gamma distribution for modeling F_1 and F_2 [72]. Other parametric choices have been described in England (1988) [79], Campbell and Ratnaparkhi (1993) [47], Walsh (1999) [281], and Sorribas et al. (2002) [251].

3.1.1.2 ROC curve estimation for the binormal model via ordinal regression: ordinal marker measurements

Diagnostic marker values are often assessed using ordinal categorical scales. This is routine practice in the assessment of imaging-based markers by human interpreters but also occurs in a variety of other clinical and laboratory settings. The structure of test data is accommodated by ordinal regression modeling [168] and can be readily implemented in most statistical software.

Because the binormal ROC curve depends only on the slope and intercept parameters defined above, an estimate of the curve can be obtained once estimates of these parameters are available. An early method for deriving estimates of the parameters for ordinal categorical test data was proposed in the seminal paper of Dorfman and Alf (1969) [69]. In an approach similar to ordinal regression, Dorfman and Alf propose to model the ordinal categorical test results as discretized values of a latent continuous variable, obtained via cut-off values, $-\infty = c_0 < c_1 \leq c_2 ... \leq c_{p-1} < c_p = \infty$, where p denotes the number of categories. For example, this variable would represent the degree of suspicion about the presence of "disease" by a test interpreter and would be elicited in a limited number of categories, usually 5 or 7. Assuming a normal distribution for the latent variable, Dorfman and Alf derived maximum likelihood estimates of the intercept and slope, while accounting for nuisance parameters. The estimates from the Dorfman and Alf method are nowadays obtained by fitting an ordinal regression model to the data, with a probit link and parameters for location and scale.

For a single marker Ytaking on values $1, 2, 3, ...C$, the general ordinal regression model has the form

$$P(Y_i \leq c|X_i) = F(\frac{\theta_c - \alpha Z_i}{exp(\beta Z_i)}), \tag{3.4}$$

for $c = 1, ..., (C-1)$. Here Y_i denotes the marker value and Z_i denotes a vector of covariates on the i-th case, F denotes a cumulative distribution function used to define the link function, α is called a *location parameter vector*, and β is called the *scale parameter vector*. Note that for $c = C$ the cumulative response probability is equal to 1.

The general ordinal regression model in Equation (3.4) with a Gaussian link can be used to fit a binormal ROC model if we specify

$$P(Y_i \leq c|X_i) = \Phi(\frac{\theta_c - \alpha X_i}{exp(\beta X_i)}),$$

with $X = 1$ if the target condition is present and $X = 0$ if the target condition is absent. The ROC parameters a, b defined in Equation (3.1) above correspond to the following functions of the parameters for the ordinal regression model: $a = \alpha \cdot exp(-\beta)$ and $b = exp(-\beta)$. Using this correspondence, the ROC curve and any quantities based on the curve, such as the AUC, can be computed from the ordinal regression model. In particular, the ROC curve can be written as the set of points

$$\{1 - \Phi(z), 1 - \Phi(exp(-\beta) \cdot z - \alpha \cdot exp(-\beta))\},$$

for $-\infty < z < \infty$ and the AUC is given by

$$AUC = \Phi(\alpha \cdot exp(-\beta)/\sqrt{1 + exp(-2\beta)}).$$

The connection with ordinal regression was a significant development in parametric ROC analysis because it made it possible to use the extensive theoretical and computational machinery of ordinal regression to derive estimates of ROC quantities. Importantly, the connection enabled regression modeling of ROC curves for single and multiple, possibly correlated, markers, and model-based methods for addressing missing data in ROC analysis [262, 263, 265]. Regression modeling of ROC curves is the topic of Chapter 6.

The function `rocfit` in `Stata` can be used to fit the binormal model for ordinal scaled data. For example, for the DMIST data presented in Table 2.7 the command `rocfit cancer ptscore if readerid==2 & modality==1 & machine==2` results in an intercept equal to $a = 0.532$ and a slope equal to $b = 0.821$, where `cancer` is the reference variable and `ptscore` is the ordinal-scaled classification variable. The respective ROC curve, produced using `rocplot`, is shown in Figure 3.4. The AUC is given by the relationship

$$AUC = \Phi(\frac{a}{\sqrt{1 + b^2}}). \tag{3.5}$$

The relevant `Stata` output follows.

```
. rocfit cancer ptscore if readerid==2 & modality==1 & machine==2

Fitting binormal model:

Iteration 0:   log likelihood = -148.31028  (not concave)
Iteration 1:   log likelihood = -145.18131  (not concave)
Iteration 2:   log likelihood = -144.83945  (not concave)
...
Iteration 16:  log likelihood = -110.96549
Iteration 17:  log likelihood = -110.96549

Binormal model of cancer on ptscore               Number of obs    =          98
Goodness-of-fit chi2(4) =         4.00
Prob > chi2             =       0.4057
Log likelihood          =   -110.96549
```

```
------------------------------------------------------------------------------
             |      Coef.   Std. Err.      z    P>|z|     [95% Conf. Interval]
-------------+----------------------------------------------------------------
   intercept |   0.531751   0.351454     1.51   0.130     -0.157087   1.220589
   slope (*) |   0.821022   0.246984    -0.72   0.469      0.336942   1.305102
-------------+----------------------------------------------------------------
       /cut1 |   0.547793   0.156286     3.51   0.000      0.241477   0.854108
       /cut2 |   0.671049   0.157861     4.25   0.000      0.361647   0.980451
       /cut3 |   1.202243   0.186060     6.46   0.000      0.837572   1.566915
       /cut4 |   1.934314   0.292543     6.61   0.000      1.360940   2.507687
       /cut5 |   2.048640   0.318011     6.44   0.000      1.425350   2.671930
       /cut6 |   2.542926   0.436601     5.82   0.000      1.687204   3.398648
------------------------------------------------------------------------------

------------------------------------------------------------------------------
             |                 Indices from binormal fit
       Index |   Estimate   Std. Err.                 [95% Conf. Interval]
-------------+----------------------------------------------------------------
    ROC area |   0.659456   0.087679                   0.487609   0.831304
    delta(m) |   0.647670   0.321828                   0.016898   1.278442
        d(e) |   0.584014   0.334882                  -0.072342   1.240370
        d(a) |   0.581214   0.338203                  -0.081652   1.244079
------------------------------------------------------------------------------
(*) z test for slope==1

. rocplot
```

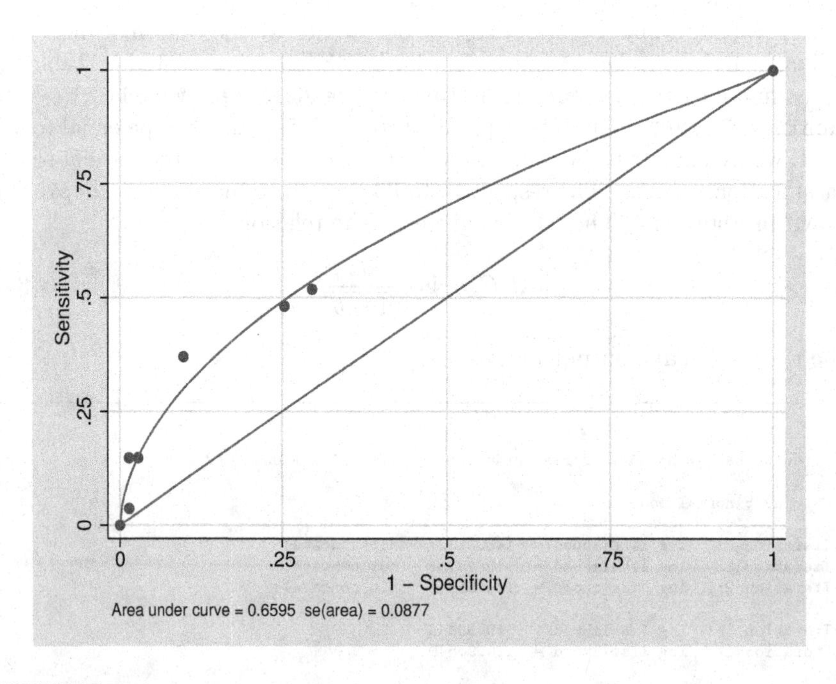

FIGURE 3.4
Smooth ROC curve based on Gaussian latent distributions for the ordinal marker measurements of Table 2.7. Points that define the empirical (1-specificity, sensitivity) pairs are also shown for reference.

Variance estimates and associated confidence intervals and regions can be obtained using the delta method. In particular, the variance of AUC can be approximated as follows:

$$Var(A\hat{U}C) = \phi(w)^2 \frac{exp(-2\hat{\beta})}{1+exp(-2\hat{\beta})}\{Var(\hat{\alpha}) - \frac{2\hat{\alpha}}{1+exp(-2\hat{\beta})} \cdot Cov(\hat{\alpha},\hat{\beta}) + \frac{\hat{\alpha}^2}{(1+exp(-2\hat{\beta}))^2} \cdot Var(\hat{\beta})\},$$

where ϕ denotes the standard normal density function, $w = \frac{\hat{\alpha} \cdot exp(-\hat{\beta})}{\sqrt{1+exp(-2\hat{\beta})}}$ and the variance and covariance terms for the estimates of α, β are obtained from the ordinal regression model.

The package `ordinal` in `R` is also suitable for this type of analysis. For the resulting location (α) and scale (β) coefficients, it still holds that, $b = e^{-\beta}$ and $a = \alpha \cdot e^{-\beta}$.

We refer the reader to the work of Ma and Hall (1993) [160] for the construction of Working-Hotelling type global, simultaneous confidence bands for the binormal ROC curve.

3.1.1.3 ROC estimation for continuous-scaled data without distributional assumptions

Metz et al. (1998) [170] present the general algorithm *LABROC4* for fitting a binormal model with continuous-scaled data without making assumptions about the distributional properties of the data. The algorithm converts the continuous measurements into categorical and then uses the Dorfman and Alf approach. As a result, the procedure is distribution-free, semi-parametric (involving likelihood-based parameter estimation), and does not require a transformation of the data to normality.

Implementation of the method is supported by `Stata`, while a useful online calculator also exists `http://www.jrocfit.org`. We illustrate the approach using the Parkinson Disease (PD) data for the diagnostic marker S-MMSE. Data of PD patients with normal cognition vs combined PD patients either with mild cognitive impairment (PD-MCI) or with dementia (PD-D) are used. Marker S-MMSE is assessed regarding its diagnostic potential in discriminating between (normal cognition) vs (MCI or Dementia) in PD patients. The estimated ROC curve is shown in Figure 3.5. The output from the `Stata` procedure includes parameter estimates for the binormal model along with indices of performance such as the AUC, just as in the ordinal marker measurements case. Notice that lower marker measurements indicate a higher severity of disease. We accommodate this fact by inverting the relevant index variable to flag with “1” patients with normal cognition.

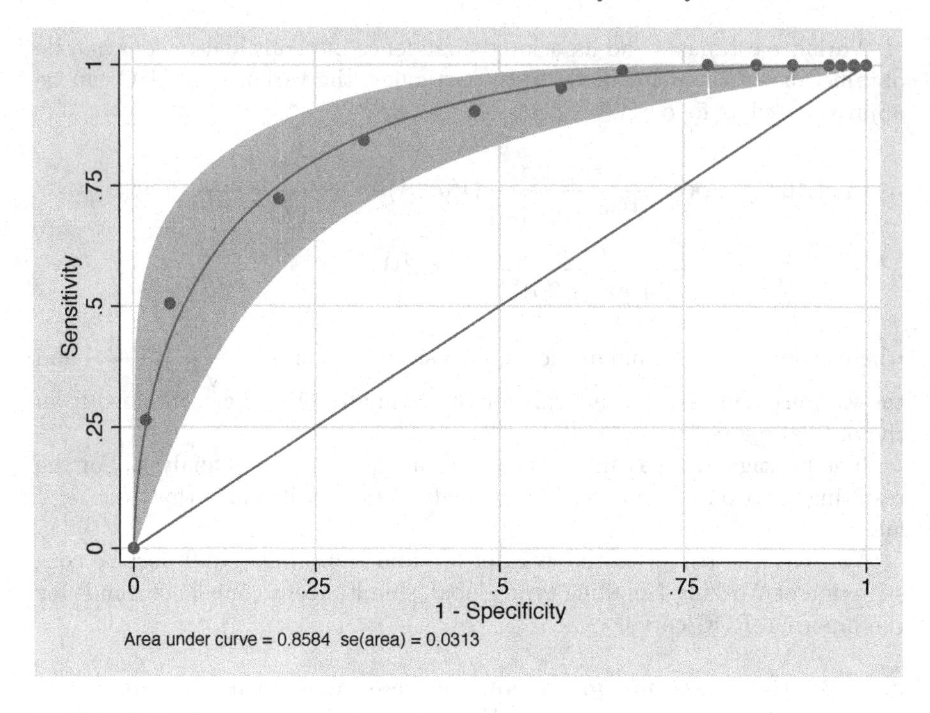

FIGURE 3.5
The semi-parametric approach for the binormal model by Metz et al. (1998) [170] for marker S-MMSE. Simultaneous 95% confidence bands are also shown.

```
. gen group=Refstd
. replace group=0 if group>=2
. quietly{
rocfit group SMMSE, continuous(.)
}
. rocplot, confband
```

3.1.1.4 Pointwise confidence bands for ROC curves derived from continuous marker data

A proper account of the uncertainty about the estimated curve needs to acknowledge the nature of the ROC curve as a two-dimensional representation of an essentially three-dimensional object involving the cut-off point on the test scale and the corresponding pairs of sensitivity and specificity. A confidence band for the curve can be constructed by considering the ensemble of the confidence regions defined by the confidence intervals for sensitivity and specificity at each value of the cut-off point. This would provide a *pointwise* confidence band for the curve, as distinct from a *global* band that accounts for uncertainty simultaneously over all cut-off points.

Assuming normal distributions for the values of the marker (appropriately transformed), each point on the ROC curve corresponds to a particular cut-off value c^* on the marker, with $sens(c) = \Phi(\frac{\mu_2 - c}{\sigma_2}) = \Phi(\delta_2)$ and $spec(c) = \Phi(\frac{c-\mu_1}{\sigma_1}) = \Phi(\delta_1)$. To obtain a $(1-\alpha)\%$ confidence interval for $sens(c^*)$, we can apply standard normal asymptotic theory on the estimate $\hat{\delta}_2 = \frac{\hat{\mu}_2 - c^*}{\hat{\sigma}_2}$, which is not bounded, and derive the interval as $\Phi(\hat{\delta}_2 \pm z_{1-\alpha/2}\sqrt{Var(\hat{\delta}_2)})$. The construction of interval for $1 - spec(c^*)$ proceeds in a similar fashion.

Since $\hat{\mu}_1$, $\hat{\mu}_2$, $\hat{\sigma}_1$, $\hat{\sigma}_2$ are all independent, using the delta method [273] we can show that,

$$Var(\hat{\delta}_2) \approx (\frac{\partial \hat{\delta}_2}{\partial \mu_1})^2 Var(\hat{\mu}_1) + (\frac{\partial \hat{\delta}_2}{\partial \sigma_1})^2 Var(\hat{\sigma}_1) + (\frac{\partial \hat{\delta}_2}{\partial \mu_2})^2 Var(\hat{\mu}_2) + (\frac{\partial \hat{\delta}_2}{\partial \sigma_2})^2 Var(\hat{\sigma}_2). \tag{3.6}$$

A similar expression can be obtained for $Var(\hat{\delta}_1)$. Estimates of the variance terms can be obtained based on $Var(\hat{\mu}_1) = \frac{\sigma_1^2}{n_1}$, $Var(\hat{\mu}_2) = \frac{\sigma_2^2}{n_2}$, $Var(\hat{\sigma}_1) = \frac{\sigma_1^2}{2(n_1-1)}$, $Var(\hat{\sigma}_2) = \frac{\sigma_2^2}{2(n_2-1)}$, as shown in Schisterman and Perkins (2007) [235].

To derive a confidence region for the ROC point, we can use a Bonferroni adjustment as follows. Note that if

$$(1 - spec_l(c^*), 1 - spec_u(c^*))$$

and

$$(sens_l(c^*), sens_u(c^*))$$

are 97.5% univariate confidence intervals for $1 - spec(c^*)$ and $sens(c^*)$, respectively, then the rectangle

$$(1 - spec_l(c^*), 1 - spec_u(c^*)) \times (sens_l(c^*), sens_u(c^*))$$

is a 95% rectangular confidence region for $(1 - spec(c^*), sens(c^*))$, where

$$sens_l(c^*) = \Phi(\hat{\delta}_2 - 2.24 \cdot \sqrt{Var(\hat{\delta}_2)}),$$

$$sens_u(c^*) = \Phi(\hat{\delta}_2 + 2.24 \cdot \sqrt{Var(\hat{\delta}_2)})$$

and similarly for $1 - spec_l(c^*)$ and $1 - spec_u(c^*)$, respectively.

The reader will note that the above construction of the confidence intervals is model-based and does not make direct use of the usual asymptotic intervals for sensitivity and specificity, based on the binomial distribution. It is well known that the latter may not be well behaved numerically and may also not have the nominal coverage [41].

3.1.2 Inference for the empirical ROC curve

A simple estimate of the ROC curve can be derived using the empirical estimators of sensitivity and specificity. The resulting *empirical* ROC curve and summary measures will suffice for descriptive analyses and can also be combined with uncertainty estimates.

The empirical ROC curve is the plot depicting $(1-\hat{F}_1(c), 1-\hat{F}_2(c)) = (\hat{S}_1(c), \hat{S}_2(c))$, for all c in the support of a diagnostic marker's measurements. Alternatively, the ROC can be written as a function of the $t = FPR$:

$$ROC(t) = S_2(S_1^{-1}(t)), \quad 0 < t < 1.$$

The corresponding empirical estimator can be derived by simply plugging- in the empirical cdfs $\hat{F}_1 = 1 - \hat{S}_1$ and $\hat{F}_2 = 1 - \hat{S}_2$ in the expression above. The variance of the empirical estimator is given by:

$$Var(\hat{ROC}(t)) = \frac{ROC(t)(1-ROC(t))}{n_2} + \left(\frac{f_2(c^*)}{f_1(c^*)}\right)^2 \times \frac{t(1-t)}{n_1}$$

where f_1 and f_2 denote the pdfs of non-diseased and diseased subjects, respectively. Note that here $c^* = S_1^{-1}(t)$. This result indicates that there are two sources of variation: the first source is from estimating the cut-off $S_1^{-1}(t)$ and is reflected in the second term of the above sum, while the second source of variation comes from the binomial variability of the estimated sensitivity when the cut-off is fixed. This is reflected by the first term of the sum above [204].

Pointwise confidence bands for the empirical ROC curve can be constructed as follows: using the notation introduced in Section 2.1.2, for a given cut-off point c^*, the empirical estimates of sensitivity and 1-specificity are

$$\hat{sens}(c^*) = \frac{\sum_{i=1}^{n_2} I(X_{2i} > c^*)}{n_2}$$

and

$$1 - \hat{spec}(c^*) = \frac{\sum_{j=1}^{n_1} I(X_{1j} > c^*)}{n_1},$$

where $I(\cdot)$ is the indicator function.

Note that the empirical estimators of sensitivity and specificity are proportions based on binomial distributions. Also, data from "diseased" and "non-diseased" cohorts are independent, so that the confidence interval for specificity is independent of that for sensitivity. Thus, if $(1-spec_l, 1-spec_u)$ and $(sens_l, sens_u)$ are 97.5% univariate confidence intervals for $1 - spec(c)$ and $sens(c)$, respectively, then the rectangle

$$(1-spec_l, 1-spec_u) \times (sens_l, sens_u)$$

is a 95% rectangular confidence region for $(1 - spec(c^*), sens(c^*))$, where

$$sens_l = \hat{sens}(c^*) - 2.24 \cdot \sqrt{\frac{\hat{sens}(c^*) \cdot (1 - \hat{sens}(c^*))}{n_2}},$$

$$sens_u = \hat{sens}(c^*) + 2.24 \cdot \sqrt{\frac{\hat{sens}(c^*) \cdot (1 - \hat{sens}(c^*))}{n_2}}$$

and similarly for $1 - spec_l$ and $1 - spec_u$.

The empirical ROC curve along with 95% pointwise confidence intervals for the S-MMSE marker for PD patients with mild cognitive impairment (PD-MCI) or dementia (PD-D) are given in Figure 3.6. The plot was constructed using the `pROC` package in `R`.

If the normal approximation to the binomial proportions is not appropriate for a specific application, the corrected Wald method that employs a logit or a probit transformation can be employed. This approach is described in Zou et al. (2013) [318].

Elliptical confidence regions for $(1 - spec(c^*), sens(c^*))$ can also be constructed in this way. In particular, a joint 95% elliptical confidence region is given by

$$\begin{bmatrix} 1 - spec - (1 - \hat{spec}(c^*)) \\ sens - \hat{sens}(c^*) \end{bmatrix} \cdot \mathbf{V}^{-1} \cdot \begin{bmatrix} 1 - spec - (1 - \hat{spec}(c^*)) \\ sens - \hat{sens}(c^*) \end{bmatrix} = q^2, \quad (3.7)$$

where q^2 is the 95% percentile of a χ^2_2 distribution and $\mathbf{V}$ is a diagonal 2×2 matrix with

$$\left(\frac{\hat{spec}(c^*) \cdot (1 - \hat{spec}(c^*))}{n_1}, \frac{\hat{sens}(c^*) \cdot (1 - \hat{sens}(c^*))}{n_2}\right)$$

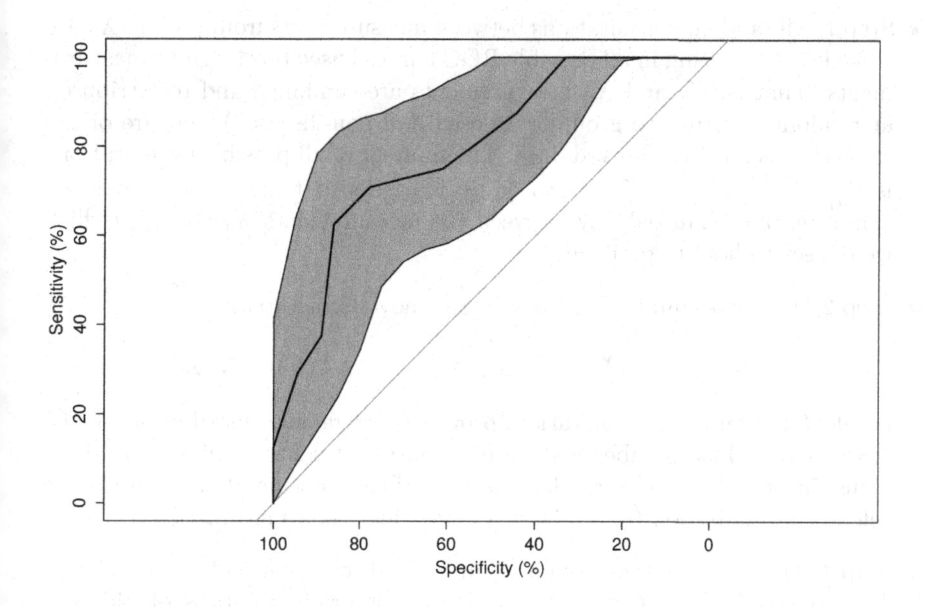

FIGURE 3.6
Empirical ROC curve along with 95% pointwise confidence intervals calculated through the `pROC` package in `R`.

in the main diagonal [142]. Construction of simultaneous confidence bands for the empirical ROC curve is more complex. The interested reader can find the details in Hsieh and Turnbull (1996) [127].

The construction of pointwise confidence intervals for the ROC curve when diagnostic marker measurements are ordinal-scaled can proceed in the same fashion as described above.

The construction of nonparametric predictive confidence intervals for the ROC curve was developed by Coolen-Maturi et al. (2012) [57]. Nonparametric predictive inference is different from the empirical method as it is explicitly predictive, considering a single next observation given the past observations, instead of aiming for inference on an entire assumed underlying population [9].

3.1.2.1 Hypothesis testing for the empirical ROC curve

A null hypothesis of interest in this context is $H_0 : F_1 = F_2$ and can be tested against $H_A : F_1 \neq F_2$ using the Kolmogorov-Smirnov (KS) two-sample statistic. The use of other than the KS statistics for the assessment of H_0 has been studied in Nakas et al. (2003) [183]. However, the KS statistic has a straightforward interpretation and is directly related to the Youden index, which is a useful summary measure in the ROC context discussed further later on.

A permutation test of the null hypothesis $H_0 : F_1 = F_2$ can be constructed as follows:

- Step 1: All random permutations between measurements from X_1 and X_2 are considered, resulting in all possible ROC curves based on the given measurements. That is, X_1 and X_2 measurements are combined and redistributed at random to form two groups (diseased and non-diseased) that are of the same size as for the observed data. The number of all possible permutations is $\frac{(n_1+n_2)!}{n_1!n_2!} = \binom{n_1+n_2}{n_1}$. This procedure is carried out under the formal assumption of exchangeability between the measurements X_1 and X_2 (which we expect to hold in practice).

- Step 2: The two-sample Kolmogorov-Smirnov (KS) statistic,

$$KS = max|X_{2i} - X_{1j}|, j = 1, \ldots, n_1, i = 1, \ldots, n_2, \tag{3.8}$$

  is calculated for each permutation, providing a reference distribution for the KS statistic. This number will be quite large even for small sample sizes. Thus, in practice, only r random permutations are generated to derive the reference distribution ($r = 1000$ is a convenient choice in practice).

- Step 3: The null hypothesis of non-significant discrimination between F_1 and F_2 is rejected when the KS statistic from the original data is outside the limits set by the 2.5% and 97.5% percentiles of the empirical distribution of the r KS statistics calculated based on the r random permutations of the original observations.

We note here that the practical utility of testing the null hypothesis of equality of the distributions of marker values seems rather limited. If H_0 is rejected, the analyst can conclude that the diagnostic marker is able to discriminate significantly between non-diseased and diseased subjects. However, the more important question is typically the magnitude of the diagnostic or predictive performance of the marker.

3.1.3 Nonparametric models

3.1.3.1 Kernel-based ROCs

Nonparametric modeling provides the means for the construction of a smooth ROC curve without making parametric assumptions about the data at hand. In particular, kernel-based smoothing has been proposed independently by Lloyd (1998) [156] and by Zou et al. (1997) [316]. We summarize here the basics of kernel density estimation needed for the material in this section. The interested reader is referred to Wand and Jones (1995) [284] for a thorough discussion of kernel density estimation.

A kernel density estimate is defined by

$$\hat{f}(x) = \frac{1}{nh} \sum_{i=1}^{n} K\left(\frac{x - X_i}{h}\right) \tag{3.9}$$

where h is a positive number known as bandwidth and $K(\cdot)$ is the kernel function that satisfies $\int K(x)dx = 1$. The kernel estimate is constructed by centering a kernel at each data point X_i, and thus the value of the kernel density estimate at a given point x is the average of the n kernel ordinates at x.

There is a variety of options regarding the choice of the kernel function. Most frequently, the kernel function is chosen to be a density function and, in particular, the Gaussian density with zero mean and standard deviation equal to one. Other kernels used in the literature include the Epanechnikov, Uniform, Triangular, Triweight, and Cosine kernel. As pointed out in Wand and Jones (1995) [284], the choice of the kernel does not appear to be of crucial importance. However, this is not the case for the choice of the bandwidth. Very small values of bandwidth would result in over-fitting while very large would result in over-smoothing.

A commonly used simple form of bandwidth is $h = (\frac{4}{3n})^{1/5}\hat{\sigma}$. To avoid the effect of outliers, Silverman's rule of thumb uses instead: $h = (\frac{4}{3n})^{1/5} min(\hat{\sigma}, IQR/1.349)$, where IQR is the inter-quartile range of the data X_i. Other options for bandwidth selection can be more data driven, based on cross validation.

The kernel-based ROC curve estimate is obtained from the kernel-based cumulative distribution functions (cdf) which is given by the equation:

$$\hat{F}(x) = \int_{-\infty}^{x} \hat{f}(t)dt. \tag{3.10}$$

If the cdf for the "non-diseased" and the "diseased" groups is denoted by $\hat{F}_1(x)$ and $\hat{F}_2(x)$, the resulting ROC curve is the plot depicting $(1 - \hat{F}_1(c), 1 - \hat{F}_2(c))$, for all c in the support of a diagnostic marker's measurements.

Zhou and Harezlak (2002) [313] compared bandwidth selection methods for kernel smoothed ROC curves. An alternative kernel choice is discussed in Zou et al. (1997) [316]. Figure 3.7 depicts the results of fitting a smooth ROC curve for the CD4 data using Gaussian kernel estimation.

A simple strategy for deriving 95% confidence intervals of either the AUC or the sensitivity (specificity) at a given specificity (sensitivity) is the use of the bootstrap. The algorithm would proceed as follows:

- Step 1: Sample with replacement from X_1 and X_2 and derive the kernels density estimates for each group separately.

- Step 2: Based on the kernel density estimates of Step 1 derive the corresponding cdf's for the current bootstrap sample.

- Step 3: Based on the cdf's of Step 2 derive the kernel-based ROC curve estimate for the current bootstrap sample. Then calculate the metric of interest (for example the AUC, denoted as $A\hat{U}C_{(b)}$ for the current bootstrap sample).

- Step 4: Repeat steps 1 and 3 $n = 1, \ldots, B$ times. Then, based on the B bootstrap samples derive the variance of the $A\hat{U}C$ by $Var(A\hat{U}C) = \frac{1}{B-1}\sum_{i=1}^{n}(A\hat{U}C_{(b)} - \bar{A\hat{U}C}_{(b)})^2$ bootstrapped values.

Using the algorithm above one may derive 95% confidence intervals by considering $\left(A\hat{U}C \pm 1.96\sqrt{Var(A\hat{U}C)}\right)$. Alternatively, confidence intervals can be constructed by first transforming the quantity of interest (here the AUC) by a logit or a probit transformation. Such intervals have the advantage that they remain within the range from 0 to 1.

The bootstrap can also be used to construct confidence intervals for other ROC metrics, such as pAUC, sensitivity at a given specificity, specificity at a given sensitivity, the Youden index etc. Those metrics will be discussed in the next sections under the empirical estimate. However, in a kernel-based framework the aforementioned algorithm can be used. For all these metrics, just as for the AUC, one can consider first transforming the metric to take values in $(-\infty, \infty)$, and then using the inverse transformation to back-transform the endpoints of the bootstrap-based confidence interval on its original scale. This will allow confidence intervals to not include values outside the unit interval $[0, 1]$.

R code for fitting a smooth ROC curve based on Gaussian kernel estimation follows. Figure 3.7 is the corresponding result. For both F_1 and F_2, $h = 4$ was set for convenience.

```
controls<-c(59, 66, 45, 62, 51, 50, 49, 58, 53, 42, 50,
47, 51, 62, 48)
cases<-c(72, 70, 69, 82, 68, 59, 76, 61, 59, 73, 49, 77)

n1<-length(controls) ; n2<-length(cases)
n<-n1+n2 ; dx<-10 ; h<-4
z<-seq(min(c(controls,cases))-dx,max(c(controls,cases))+dx)
m1<-matrix(0,n,length(z)) ; m2<-matrix(0,n,length(z))

for (i in 1:n1) {m1[i,]<-dnorm(z,controls[i],h)}
for (j in 1:n2) {m2[j,]<-dnorm(z,cases[j],h)}

zfreq1<-apply(m1,2,sum) ; zfreq2<-apply(m2,2,sum)

par(mfrow=c(1,2))
plot(z,zfreq1,xlab="CD4 counts",ylab="Densities",
xlim=c(20,100),ylim=c(0,1),type="l", lty=1)
par(new=T)
plot(z,zfreq2,type="l",lty=2,xlim=c(20,100),ylim=c(0,1),
xlab="",ylab="")
legend(20,1,c("Controls","Cases"),lty=c(seq(1,2)))

on<-sort(c(controls,cases))
FP<-NULL ; TP<-NULL

grille<-c(on-1,on)
for (i in 1:length(grille)){
  one<-controls[controls>=grille[i]]
  two<-cases[cases>=grille[i]]
  FP[i]<-length(one)/length(controls)
  TP[i]<-length(two)/length(cases)
}

FP1<-NULL ; TP1<-NULL
one1<-NULL ; two1<-NULL
lz<-length(z)

for (i in 1:lz){
  one1[i]<-sum(zfreq1[i:lz])
  two1[i]<-sum(zfreq2[i:lz])}

FP1<-one1/sum(zfreq1)
TP1<-two1/sum(zfreq2)
```

```
plot(FP,TP,xlab="1-Specificity",ylab="Sensitivity",
xlim=c(0,1),ylim=c(0,1))
par(new=T)
plot(FP1,TP1,xlab="",ylab="",type="l",xlim=c(0,1),
ylim=c(0,1))
```

3.1.3.2 Spline-based ROCs

A spline is a piecewise polynomial model that is usually met under a regression framework. Regression splines are piecewise polynomials and are often an appealing modeling strategy due to their flexibility [237]. The process of fitting a spline starts by considering a set of knots (points on the x-axis). For each consecutive pair of knots, a polynomial is fitted under some conditions of continuity so that the whole spline function is a continuous function for the full range of support. Splines can also be employed for other settings, such as density estimation, and as a result ROC curve estimation. A spline model can be an alternative approach of obtaining a smooth ROC estimate. As has already been discussed, knowledge of the two underlying densities of the two

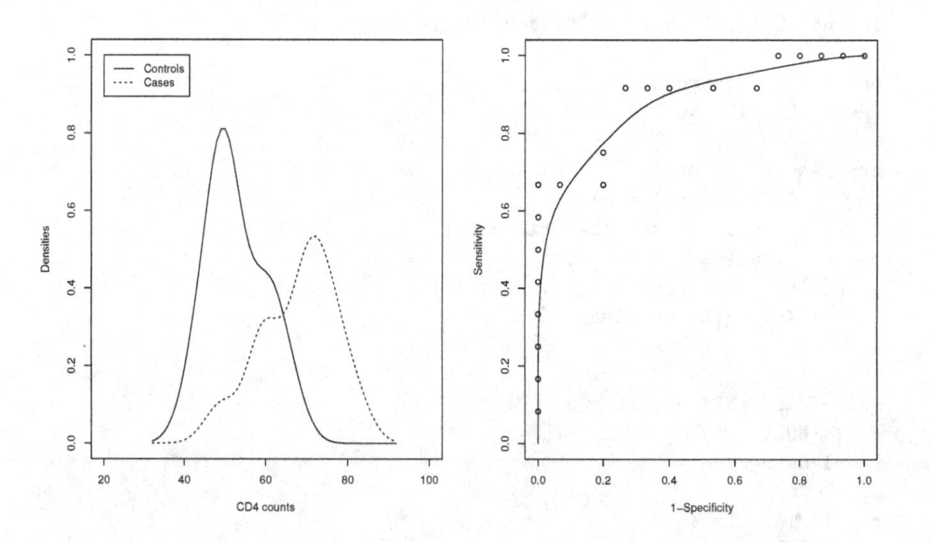

FIGURE 3.7
Smooth ROC curve based on Gaussian kernel smoothing for the CD4 data. Points that define the empirical (1-specificity, sensitivity) pairs are also shown for reference.

groups ("non-diseased" vs "diseased") allows for the construction of the ROC curve. Equivalently, knowledge of the corresponding cumulative distribution functions (cdfs), or the cumulative hazard functions ($H(x) = -log(S(x))$), allows for the construction of the ROC curve. Below we discuss two spline-based approaches, through which one can obtain a smooth estimate of $S(x) = 1 - F(x) = 1 - \int_{-\infty}^{x} f(t)dt$ for each of the two groups (separately). An ROC curve can then be constructed by using:

$$ROC(\cdot) = \{(S_1(c), S_2(c)), -\infty < c < \infty\}.$$

We start with the so-called logspline approach that has been employed to derive an ROC curve. The logspline was initially presented by Kooperberg and Stone (1992) [139] under a density estimation framework. Consider K knots, with $K \geq 3$, denoted by the sequence $\tau_1, \ldots, \tau_K$ with $-\infty \leq L < \tau_1 < \ldots < \tau_K \leq U \leq \infty$, where L and U are numbers that define the support of the marker measurements. The logspline density model of the biomarker scores for any of the two groups is considered to be:

$$f(x;\theta) = exp(\theta_1 B_1(x) + \ldots + \theta_p B_p(x) - C(\theta)), \quad L < x < U, \tag{3.11}$$

where

$$C(\theta) = log(\int_L^U exp(\theta_1 B_1(x) + \ldots + \theta_p B_p(x))dx)$$

is the normalizing constant, $\theta = (\theta_1, \ldots, \theta_p)$ are the unknown spline parameters to be estimated and $B_1(x)$, $B_2(x)$,..., $B_p(x)$ are the spline basis functions. These can appropriately be defined in order to form a natural cubic spline for which the condition

$$\int_L^U exp(\theta_1 B_1(x) + \ldots + \theta_p B_p(x))dx < \infty$$

is satisfied. The corresponding logspline survival function is then given by

$$S(x;\theta) = 1 - \int_L^x f(z,\theta)dz, \quad L < x < U.$$

The estimate is based on maximum likelihood and the process when estimating the underlying ROC involves fitting the logspline model separately for the measurements of diseased and non-diseased subjects. Using these densities, we can easily derive the corresponding survival functions for each group namely $\hat{S}_{X_1}(\cdot)$ and $\hat{S}_{X_2}(\cdot)$. The smooth logspline-based ROC curve is then defined by:

$$\hat{ROC}(\cdot) = \{(\hat{S}_1(c), \hat{S}_2(c)), -\infty < c < \infty\}.$$

Inferences around the metrics of interest can be based on the bootstrap in a similar fashion as was previously described.

The Hazard Constrained Natural Spline (HCNS) [21], which was introduced in a survival analysis context and was further developed for ROC analysis [17] is presented next. Consider K distinct knots $\tau_1 < \tau_2 < \cdots < \tau_K$.

Denote $x_+ = \max(0, x)$ and consider the following model for the cumulative hazard function:

$$
\begin{aligned}
H(x) = {} & \beta_1(x-\tau_1)_+^3 + \cdots + \beta_{K-2}(x-\tau_{K-2})_+^3 + \beta_{K-1}(x-\tau_{K-1})_+^3 \\
& + \beta_K(x-\tau_K)_+^3
\end{aligned}
\tag{3.12}
$$

where

$$
\beta_{K-1} = \frac{\beta_1(\tau_1-\tau_K) + \beta_2(\tau_2-\tau_K) + \cdots + \beta_{K-2}(\tau_{K-2}-\tau_K)}{\tau_K - \tau_{K-1}} \tag{3.13}
$$

$$
\beta_K = \frac{\beta_1(\tau_1-\tau_{K-1}) + \beta_2(\tau_2-\tau_{K-1}) + \cdots + \beta_{K-2}(\tau_{K-2}-\tau_{K-1})}{\tau_{K-1} - \tau_K}
$$

The model from Equation (3.12) has the following properties [22, 23]:

1. It is linear beyond the last knot;
2. It equals zero before the first knot;
3. Its first and second derivatives are continuous;
4. Its first derivative is zero at the first knot; and
5. It has $K-2$ parameters to be estimated.

ROC curve estimation is done in two steps. In the first step, the underlying survival function of each group is derived through the empirical estimate. In the second step, the model from Equation (3.12) is fitted to the corners of the cumulative step empirical hazard function. However, the cumulative hazard function is monotone, and thus monotonicity restrictions must be imposed. These can be linear as done in Bantis et al. (2012) [21]. The objective function to minimize is the distance of the spline-based form of the cumulative hazard from the corners of the stepwise estimate of the cumulative hazard ($\hat{H}^{emp}$). That is:

$$
\Psi(\hat{\beta}) = \sum_i \left(\hat{H}(X_i) - \hat{H}^{emp}(X_i) \right)^2 \tag{3.14}
$$

under some linear constraints of monotonicity. Thus, the problem is a restricted least squares one, with linear restrictions on the parameters. Hence, convergence is guaranteed since the function to minimize is always convex.

Note that this approach does not involve any likelihood maximization once the empirical estimates of the cumulative hazard are obtained for each group. Regarding the knot placement different schemes could be employed. A robust strategy is the following [23]: Derive 10 equally spaced points that expand from min(scores) $= \min(X_i)$ up to max(scores) $= \max(X_i)$; each of these points is a candidate for placing a knot. Using 6 knots, there are $10!/(6!4!) = 210$ possible combinations, and thus 210 possible knot schemes. Next, we consider 10 points at the following percentiles that are calculated only by the fully observed data: $0, 2.5^{th}$, 5th, 10th, 20th, 40th, 50th, 60th, 80th, and 100th percentiles. Exploring again all possible combinations, there are 210 additional combinations (knot schemes) to be explored.

In a given application, all 420 knot schemes are tested by fitting the model of Equation (3.12) to the empirical-based cumulative hazard function. Finally, the knot scheme that results in the smallest distance to the corners of the step function is chosen. The same process is repeated for both groups separately. This may seem like a difficult task from the point of view of computing time. However, with current computer technology, this procedure is only a matter of seconds. In effect, resampling methods are feasible for statistical inference on a given data set, as previously presented through the bootstrap. A full package that applies the HCNS as well as bootstrap-based inferences is provided in `leobantis.net`.

In spite of these smoothing techniques, both spline- and kernel-based, the vast majority of the clinical literature relies on the empirical-based ROC estimate. However, there are several arguments in favor of the smoothing estimates. First, the true and generally unknown ROC curve is usually supposed to be smooth and it seems unnatural for its estimate to not share that property. Lloyd and Yong (1999) [157] show the superiority of a kernel based ROC over the empirical ROC estimate through rates of convergence. Having a smooth ROC estimate comes with additional computational advantages as it is differentiable, an important property that is also useful in calculating the variability $Var(\hat{ROC}(t))$ at any given t.

Pointwise confidence intervals for the ROC curve after nonparametric modelling can be constructed in the same way as in the empirical case discussed in Section 3.1.2. Theoretical justifications are discussed in depth in Hall et al. (2004) [101].

Other ROC curve smoothing approaches involve the use of Bernstein polynomials [287], while Bayesian nonparametric modeling has been developed by Hanson et al. (2008) [106] and by Branscum et al. (2008) [39].

Some basic ROC curve models

For a diagnostic marker with continuous-scaled measurements

- Empirical model: $(\frac{\sum_{j=1}^{n_1} I(X_{1j}>c)}{n_1}, \frac{\sum_{i=1}^{n_2} I(X_{2i}>c)}{n_2})$, for all c. $I(\cdot)$ is the indicator function. Empirical estimates of the survival function such as the Kaplan-Meier estimate can be used.

- Binormal model (parametric): $ROC(t) = \Phi(\frac{\mu_2-\mu_1+\sigma_1\Phi^{-1}(t)}{\sigma_2})$, $t \in [0,1]$. The binormal model can be used directly if parametric assumptions are met, after applying the Box-Cox transformation, or using the LABROC4 algorithm by Metz et al. (1998) [170].

- Kernel smoothed (nonparametric): $(1 - \hat{F}_1(t), 1 - \hat{F}_2(t))$, with $\hat{F}_i(t) = \frac{1}{n_i}\Sigma_{j=1}^{n_i}\Phi(\frac{t-X_{ij}}{h_i})$, $i = 1,2$ and $h_i = (\frac{4}{3n_i})^{1/5} min(\hat{\sigma}_i, IQR_i/1.349)$.

For a diagnostic marker with ordinal-scaled measurements

- Empirical model: Same as above.
- Binormal model (parametric): Use `rocfit` with `Stata` or `clm` from package `ordinal` with `R`.

3.2 Inference for ROC Summary Measures

Summaries of the ROC curve such as the full or the partial Area Under the ROC Curve and the maximum of the Youden index capture salient aspects of the information provided by the ROC curve in relatively simple, quantitative, and interpretable measures. These summary measures, rather than the full curve, are typically used to draw conclusions in empirical studies. In this section we discuss properties of the summary measures of the ROC curve and present methods for drawing statistical inference.

The AUC was introduced in Section 2.2.3.1. It is the standard single measure reported in the scientific literature for the assessment of the diagnostic performance of a marker. The AUC can be interpreted as the average sensitivity for all values of specificity and, at the same time, the average specificity for all values of sensitivity. Its importance as a measure of performance is aided greatly by the fact that it has an intuitive interpretation: for a randomly chosen pair of subjects comprising one from the non-diseased and one from the diseased population, the AUC is the probability that the measurement from the non-diseased subject will be less than the measurement from the diseased subject, or $AUC = P(X_1 < X_2)$ for continuous markers.

The maximum of the Youden index of a marker, defined as

$$J = max_c\{sens(c) + spec(c) - 1\} = max_c|F_1(c) - F_2(c)|,$$

is the maximum distance from the ROC curve to the main diagonal line in the unit square. The points on this line satisfy the relation $sens = 1 - spec$. The maximum of Youden index is typically used to derive an optimal cut-off point for making decisions on the basis of the marker.

3.2.1 Statistical inference for the AUC

3.2.1.1 Nonparametric methods

The AUC is estimated nonparametrically as

$$\hat{AUC} = \frac{1}{n_1 n_2} \sum_{j=1}^{n_1} \sum_{i=1}^{n_2} [I(X_{2i} > X_{1j}) + \frac{1}{2} \cdot I(X_{2i} = X_{1j})], \quad (3.15)$$

where $I(\cdot)$ is the indicator function, with $I(\mathcal{A}) = 1$ if $\mathcal{A}$ is true (otherwise it is equal to zero).

The expression in Equation (3.15) is equivalent to the Wilcoxon–Mann–Whitney statistic (Chapter 4 in Zhou et al. (2011) [314]). As a result, properties of the Wilcoxon–Mann–Whitney statistic can also be used in inference for the AUC (see e.g. Lehmann and D'Abrera (2006) [145]).

To construct confidence intervals for the AUC, an estimate of its variance is needed. A variety of strategies have been proposed in the literature for the estimation of $Var(AUC)$.

The standard nonparametric approach can be found in De Long et al. (1988) [64] and is based on U-statistics theory [123]:

$$Var(\hat{AUC}) = \frac{1}{n_1(n_1-1)} \sum_{j=1}^{n_1} (D_{10}(X_{1j}) - \hat{AUC})^2 + \frac{1}{n_2(n_2-1)} \sum_{i=1}^{n_2} (D_{01}(X_{2i}) - \hat{AUC})^2, \quad (3.16)$$

where

$$D_{10}(X_{1j}) = \frac{1}{n_2} \sum_{i=1}^{n_2} [I(X_{2i} > X_{1j}) + \frac{1}{2} \cdot I(X_{2i} = X_{1j})]$$

and

$$D_{01}(X_{2i}) = \frac{1}{n_1} \sum_{j=1}^{n_1} [I(X_{2i} > X_{1j}) + \frac{1}{2} \cdot I(X_{2i} = X_{1j})].$$

A 95% confidence interval for the AUC is given by

$$(\hat{AUC} - 1.96 \cdot \sqrt{Var(\hat{AUC})}, \hat{AUC} + 1.96 \cdot \sqrt{Var(\hat{AUC})}). \quad (3.17)$$

In an earlier paper, Hanley and McNeil (1982) [105] offered a simple closed-form expression for $Var(AUC)$ estimation for the empirical and the nonparametric cases:

$$\begin{aligned} Var(\hat{AUC}) = \frac{1}{n_1 n_2}(AUC(1 - AUC) + (n_1 - 1)(Q_1 - AUC^2) \\ + (n_2 - 1)(Q_2 - AUC^2)), \end{aligned} \quad (3.18)$$

where Q_1 is the probability that marker values of two randomly chosen "diseased" subjects are larger than the marker value of a randomly chosen "non-diseased" subject, and Q_2 is the probability that the marker value of one randomly chosen "diseased" subject is larger than the marker values of two randomly chosen "non-diseased" subjects. In practice these quantities are not easy to estimate for a general distribution. However, simple estimates are available under the assumption of an exponential distribution for the marker. In this case, $Q_1 = \frac{AUC}{2-AUC}$ and $Q_2 = \frac{2AUC^2}{1+AUC}$.

Closed-form expressions for the variance are useful for design and sample size considerations as discussed in Section 4.5. However, the simple estimator may perform poorly in some settings as shown by Newcombe (2006) [192], and Qin and Hotilovac (2008) [216], who compared several different approaches for the estimation of confidence intervals for AUC in the nonparametric case.

3.2.1.2 Parametric methods

A parametric estimate of the AUC can be obtained from the binormal model by using the formula $AUC = \Phi(\frac{\mu_2-\mu_1}{\sqrt{\sigma_2^2+\sigma_1^2}})$ that can be derived from the functional form of the ROC curve by integrating the corresponding function over $[0,1]$. To estimate the AUC parametrically, we simply plug-in the usual estimators for mean and variance. As a result,

$$A\hat{U}C = \Phi(\frac{\hat{\mu}_2 - \hat{\mu}_1}{\sqrt{\hat{\sigma}_2^2 + \hat{\sigma}_1^2}}) \tag{3.19}$$

is used in practice. Equation (3.19) offers a closed form expression for the AUC which can be very useful in practice for computational purposes.

The delta method has been used to construct confidence intervals for AUC under the binormal model [166, 289, 318]. Specifically, let $\delta = \frac{\mu_2-\mu_1}{\sqrt{\sigma_2^2+\sigma_1^2}}$ and $\hat{\delta}$ the respective estimator of δ based on $\hat{\mu}_1, \hat{\mu}_2, \hat{\sigma}_1, \hat{\sigma}_2$.

Then,

$$Var(\hat{\delta}) \approx (\frac{\partial\delta}{\partial\mu_1})^2 Var(\hat{\mu}_1) + (\frac{\partial\delta}{\partial\sigma_1})^2 Var(\hat{\sigma}_1) + (\frac{\partial\delta}{\partial\mu_2})^2 Var(\hat{\mu}_2) + (\frac{\partial\delta}{\partial\sigma_2})^2 Var(\hat{\sigma}_2). \tag{3.20}$$

A 95% confidence interval for AUC is given by

$$(\Phi(\hat{\delta} - 1.96 \cdot \sqrt{Var(\hat{\delta})}), \Phi(\hat{\delta} + 1.96 \cdot \sqrt{Var(\hat{\delta})})). \tag{3.21}$$

The variance of the AUC estimate given in Equation (3.19) can also be estimated as

$$\begin{aligned} Var(A\hat{U}C) \approx (\frac{\partial A\hat{U}C}{\partial\mu_1})^2 Var(\hat{\mu}_1) + (\frac{\partial A\hat{U}C}{\partial\sigma_1})^2 Var(\hat{\sigma}_1) + (\frac{\partial A\hat{U}C}{\partial\mu_2})^2 Var(\hat{\mu}_2) \\ + (\frac{\partial A\hat{U}C}{\partial\sigma_2})^2 Var(\hat{\sigma}_2). \end{aligned} \tag{3.22}$$

A drawback for this approach is that the confidence interval for the AUC may exceed the $[0,1]$ limits. This is similar to the performance of Wald estimates for binomial proportions. To avoid this problem, we recommend the use of the confidence interval given in Equation (3.21).

Symbolic programming can be used for the implementation of the above procedures. A relevant `R` function is given below. Alternative approaches for inference for the AUC under binormality using approximate methods are described in Reiser and Guttman (1986) [220]. The latter have not been widely used in practice so far.

`R` code for the construction of 95% confidence intervals for AUC using the delta method follows.

```
x<-c(59, 66, 45, 62, 51, 50, 49, 58, 53, 42, 50, 47,
 51, 62, 48)
y<-c(72, 70, 69, 82, 68, 59, 76, 61, 59, 73, 49, 77)

aucsi<-function(x,y){

mu1<-mean(x) ; mu2<-mean(y)
si1<-sd(x) ;  si2<-sd(y)
n1<-length(x) ; n2<-length(y)

auc<-pnorm((mu2-mu1)/sqrt(si1^2+si2^2))

alpha<-expression((m2-m1)/sqrt(s1^2+s2^2))
alph1<-D(alpha,"m1")
alpha1<-eval(alph1, list(s1=si1, s2=si2))
alph2<-D(alpha,"m2")
alpha2<-eval(alph2, list(s1=si1, s2=si2))

bet1<-D(alpha,"s1")
beta1<-eval(bet1, list(s1=si1, s2=si2, m1=mu1,m2=mu2))
bet2<-D(alpha,"s2")
beta2<-eval(bet2, list(s1=si1, s2=si2, m1=mu1,m2=mu2))

varfauc<-alpha1^2*(si1^2/n1)+beta1^2*(si1^2/(2*n1-2))+
alpha2^2*(si2^2/n2)+beta2^2*(si2^2/(2*n2-2))

aucest<-(mu2-mu1)/sqrt(si1^2+si2^2)
auclb<-pnorm(aucest-1.96*sqrt(varfauc))
aucub<-pnorm(aucest+1.96*sqrt(varfauc))

return(list(auc,auclb,aucub))
}
aucsi(x,y)
```

```
## [[1]]
```

```
## [1] 0.9017913
##
## [[2]]
## [1] 0.7335023
##
## [[3]]
## [1] 0.9750145
```

3.2.1.3 Bootstrap-based inference for AUC

A bootstrap approach can also be used for the estimation of $Var(AUC)$ or for the direct construction of confidence intervals for AUC. The bootstrap approach can be adapted for use with all different models and has been shown to perform very well in many settings [216]. In fact, the bootstrap paradigm can always be used in practice as an easy-to-implement approach, yet, occasionally computationally intensive, for the estimation of the variance of a parameter of interest or for the direct estimation of confidence intervals thereof.

A basic bootstrap algorithm for the construction of confidence intervals proceeds along the following steps,

- Step 1: Measurements from X_1 and from X_2 are sampled independently with replacement b times.
- Step 2: AUC is calculated for each of the b bootstrap replications ($b = 2000$ is a convenient choice).
- Step 3: The resulting AUC replications are ordered and the 2.5% and 97.5% quantiles of the resulting AUC bootstrap distribution define the 95% confidence interval for AUC.

Many different variants of this algorithm can be considered. In particular, the AUC can be calculated in Step 2 either empirically or parametrically. For example, under the binormal model, one can estimate a, b, either directly from the data or after some normalizing transformation. Another option is to estimate the sample variance directly from the b bootstrap $AUCs$ and use this for inference (see e.g. Davison and Hinkley (1997) [63]). The different options will yield slightly different results depending on the distributional properties of the initial marker measurements. The package `pROC` makes heavy use of bootstrap methods for inference within the ROC curve framework. Implementation of bootstrap algorithms using base `R` or the `boot` package is also an option.

We provide here `R` code for the construction of confidence intervals for the AUC based on bootstrap. The code produces 95% confidence intervals for the AUC based on the CD4 data using $b = 1000$ bootstrap replicates. In this example, the AUC is estimated empirically.

```
controls<-c(59, 66, 45, 62, 51, 50, 49, 58, 53, 42, 50,
47, 51, 62, 48)
cases<-c(72, 70, 69, 82, 68, 59, 76, 61, 59, 73, 49, 77)

n.con<-length(controls)
n.cas<-length(cases)
auc<-rep(0,1000)

for (j in 1:1000){
cont<-sample(controls, replace=T)
case<-sample(cases, replace=T)
subj<-unique(sort(c(cont,case)))
subj.con<-unique(sort(cont))
subj.cas<-unique(sort(case))
n.tot<-length(subj)

tp<-rep(0,n.tot) ; fp<-rep(0,n.tot)

for (i in 1:n.tot){
  tp[i]<-sum(case >= subj[i])/n.cas
  fp[i]<-sum(cont >= subj[i])/n.con
}
tp<-c(1,tp,0) ; fp<-c(1,fp,0)

tp.mean<-(tp[1:(n.tot+1)] + tp[2:(n.tot+2)])/2
fp.diff<--diff(fp)
auc[j]<-sum(fp.diff*tp.mean)
}

auc<-sort(auc)
#auc
auc[25]
auc[975]
```

```
## > auc[25]
## [1] 0.7361111
## > auc[975]
## [1] 0.9888889
```

3.2.2 Hypothesis testing for AUC

So far in this chapter we have focused on inference based on point estimates for the AUC, followed by the construction of corresponding 95% confidence intervals. These intervals can be used to assess specific hypotheses of interest for the AUC. For example, if the confidence interval does not include 0.5, one may conclude that the marker under study significantly separates between controls and cases.

Formal hypothesis testing would begin by specifying a null hypothesis, for example, $H_0 : AUC = 0.5$ and an alternative hypothesis, for example, $H_A : AUC \neq 0.5$. A one- or a two-sided test can be based on the test statistic,

$$Z = \frac{\hat{AUC} - 0.5}{\sqrt{Var(\hat{AUC})}}. \tag{3.23}$$

Z follows approximately a standard normal distribution under the null hypothesis [127, 143]. The corresponding one- or two-sided p-value can then be computed.

The following simple R code implements Equation (3.23) using the pROC package for the estimation of the variance of the AUC using Equation (3.16). Based on the corresponding output, one concludes that CD4 may have promise as a biomarker for the detection of brucellosis $AUC = 0.886$, (95% CI:0.752, 1.000), $p < 0.001$.

```
library(pROC)

brucon<-c(59, 66, 45, 62, 51, 50, 49, 58, 53, 42, 50, 47, 51, 62, 48)
brucas<-c(72, 70, 69, 82, 68, 59, 76, 61, 59, 73, 49, 77)

cd4roc<-roc(controls=brucon, cases=brucas)

auc(cd4roc)
ci(auc(cd4roc))
2*(1-pnorm((auc(cd4roc)-0.5)/sqrt(var(auc(cd4roc)))))
#two-sided test
```

```
## > auc(cd4roc)
## Area under the curve: 0.8861
## > ci(auc(cd4roc))
## 95% CI: 0.7523-1 (DeLong)
## > 2*(1-pnorm((auc(cd4roc)-0.5)/sqrt(var(auc(cd4roc)))))
## [1] 1.55205e-08
```

Permutation tests can also be constructed for the AUC. As an example, for the simple hypothesis $H_0 : AUC = 0.5$ discussed in this section, a p-value can be derived as follows:

- Step 1: Measurements from X_1 and X_2 are combined in a single vector forming a set of $n_1 + n_2$ measurements.

- Step 2: All random permutations of the single, combined vector are considered. In practice a convenient number of r permutations (e.g. $r = 1000$) are used.
- Step 3: For each permutation, the first n_1 measurements are considered as arising from X_1 and the rest n_2 as arising from X_2.
- Step 4: For each permutation the corresponding AUC is calculated. As a result, a sample of r AUCs, $(AUC_1^p, \ldots, AUC_r^p)$ is derived.
- Step 5: The p-value corresponding to evaluating H_0 is the proportion of AUC^r that are larger than the AUC calculated from the original data.

The permutation testing approach can also be used, along with the bootstrap, for all different models described earlier. The validity of the Z-score in Equation (3.23), strictly speaking, depends on the estimates of the variance in the denominator, although it is expected to perform adequately well in practice.

Basic inference for AUC

For a diagnostic marker with continuous-scaled measurements,

- Empirical and nonparametric AUC estimator:

$$\hat{AUC} = \frac{1}{n_1 n_2} \sum_{j=1}^{n_1} \sum_{i=1}^{n_2} [I(X_{2i} > X_{1j}) + \frac{1}{2} I(X_{2i} = X_{1j})].$$

  $I(\cdot)$ is the indicator function. Use U-statistics theory or the bootstrap for $Var(\hat{AUC})$ estimation.

- Binormal AUC estimator:

$$\hat{AUC} = \Phi(\frac{\hat{\mu}_2 - \hat{\mu}_1}{\sqrt{\hat{\sigma}_2^2 + \hat{\sigma}_1^2}}).$$

  Use delta method or the bootstrap for $Var(\hat{AUC})$ estimation.

- Hypothesis testing for $H_0 : AUC = 0.5$: $Z = \frac{AUC - 0.5}{\sqrt{Var(AUC)}} \sim N(0, 1)$. A permutation testing approach can be used instead.

3.2.3 Statistical inference for the partial Area Under the ROC Curve (pAUC)

The partial area under the ROC curve (pAUC) was introduced in the previous chapter (Section 2.2.3.1) as a measure of marker performance when only a range of sensitivity or specificity is of practical interest. For example, in the case of markers used in screening, high values of specificity are of practical interest. Sometimes, interest may focus on a range of specificities and their corresponding sensitivities (or vice versa), say from measurement c_a to measurement c_b thus defining a clinically relevant portion of the ROC curve instead of the whole curve. If that is the case, estimation of the respective partial AUC (pAUC) is of interest which is formally defined by

$$pAUC(c_a, c_b) = \int_{c_a}^{c_b} ROC(c)dc.$$

The pAUC has bounds that are tighter than $[0, 1]$, specifically

$$\frac{1}{2}(c_b - c_a) \cdot (c_b + c_a) \leq pAUC \leq (c_b - c_a). \tag{3.24}$$

Calculation of $Var(pAUC)$ based on the delta method can be done in pretty much the same way as for AUC. The basic theory is described in McClish (1989) [166]. A nonparametric and a bootstrap alternative are offered with the R package `pROC`. The latter package offers the possibility to estimate the ROC curve, the AUC and partial AUC, provides confidence intervals for all estimated quantities and has nice graphing choices. Results of the `pROC` package using the PD data for the diagnostic marker S-MMSE are illustrated in Figure 3.8. Data of PD patients with mild cognitive impairment (PD-MCI) vs PD patients with dementia (PD-D) are used. Marker S-MMSE is assessed regarding its diagnostic potential in discriminating between MCI and Dementia in PD patients. Restricting the analysis to the range of sensitivities between 0.8 and 1, we obtain $pAUC = 0.682$, (95% CI: $0.597, 0.788$).

The fact that pAUC restricts attention to a region of specificity (or sensitivity) rather than the entire interval [0,1] has intuitive appeal in many research settings [67].

3.2.4 Selection of optimal points and cut-offs, Youden index

Once the diagnostic accuracy of the marker is established, the selection of an optimal cut-off point is needed which will be used by practitioners for screening purposes. The cut-off point must be selected based on an optimality criterion. The maximum of the Youden index is used in practice quite often because of its simplicity. The empirical estimator of the maximum of the Youden index is defined as

$$J = max_c\{\hat{sens}(c) + \hat{spec}(c) - 1\} = max_c|\hat{F}_1(c) - \hat{F}_2(c)| \tag{3.25}$$

and it is equivalent to the (KS) statistic, given in Equation (3.8). Inference for the ROC curve based on the empirical estimator of the maximum of the Youden index follows from this equivalence. The procedure is described in detail in Gail and Green (1976) [90].

The relative importance of sensitivity and specificity for any given problem can be reflected in the choice of the optimal cut-off point by introducing

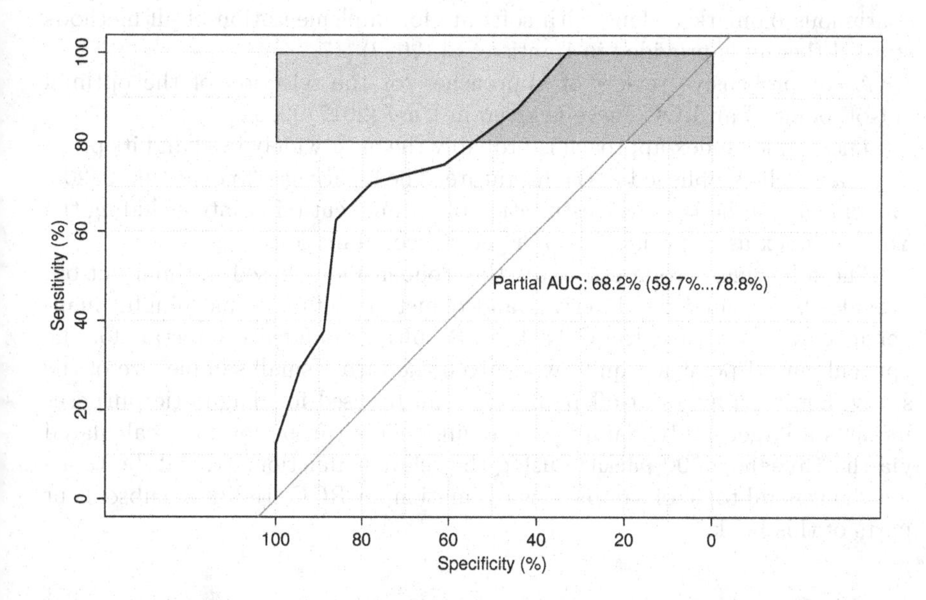

FIGURE 3.8
Empirical ROC curve along with 95% pointwise confidence intervals for a relevant range of sensitivities calculated through the pROC package in R.

weights, ν and μ, in the general definition of the maximum of the Youden index as follows: $J^* = max_c\{\nu \cdot sens(c) + \mu \cdot spec(c) - 1\}$. In practice, these weights can be difficult to set [98].

Under the assumption that marker values for non-diseased and diseased subjects follow normal distributions $N(\mu_1, \sigma_1^2)$ and $N(\mu_2, \sigma_2^2)$, respectively, the maximum of the Youden index is defined as

$$J = max_c\{\Phi(\frac{c - \mu_1}{\sigma_1}) + \Phi(\frac{\mu_2 - c}{\sigma_2}) - 1\} \tag{3.26}$$

and the corresponding optimal cut-off point, c^*, has the following closed-form expression,

$$c^* = \frac{\sigma_1^2\mu_2 - \sigma_2^2\mu_1 - \sigma_1\sigma_2\sqrt{(\mu_1 - \mu_2)^2 + (\sigma_1^2 - \sigma_2^2)\log(\frac{\sigma_1^2}{\sigma_2^2})}}{\sigma_1^2 - \sigma_2^2}, \text{ if } \sigma_1 \neq \sigma_2. \tag{3.27}$$

Otherwise, $c^* = \frac{\mu_1+\mu_2}{2}$. J, c^* and other parameters of interest are estimated by substituting for the unknown μ_1, μ_2, σ_1, σ_2 in the above formulae the corresponding sample means and standard deviations. Estimation of $Var(\hat{c}^*)$ and $Var(\hat{J})$ using the delta method has been developed by Schisterman and Perkins (2007) [235].

An in-depth treatment of the construction of confidence intervals for the maximum of the Youden index and the corresponding cut-off point of a continuous biomarker along with software for implementation of all methods studied therein is provided in Bantis et al (2019) [17].

A comprehensive review of approaches for the selection of the optimal cut-off point of an ROC curve is given in Unal (2017) [269].

The Youden index approach is probably the most widely used and its properties are well-established in the literature. The `R` package `ThresholdROC` [206] implements methods for the estimation of optimal cut-off points including the Youden index as a special case of a general cost function.

The following `R` code estimates the Youden index-based optimal cut-off, provides 95% confidence intervals and depicts results in a meaningful manner in Figure 3.9 using the CD4 data. Resulting confidence intervals for the optimal cut-off point are quite wide given the rather small sample size of the study. Establishing a cut-off point that can be used for diagnostic purposes requires a larger study. Sample size requirements can be formally calculated via the `ThresholdROC` package using the relevant function. We will be treating the general topic of sample size estimation for ROC studies in subsequent parts of this book.

```
library(ThresholdROC)

controls<-c(59, 66, 45, 62, 51, 50, 49, 58, 53, 42, 50,
            47, 51, 62, 48)
cases<-c(72, 70, 69, 82, 68, 59, 76, 61, 59, 73, 49, 77)

cutyi<-thres2(controls, cases, rho=0.5, method="empirical",
  ci.method = "boot")
cutyi
plot(cutyi)
```

```
## Estimate:
##  Threshold:  68
##  Minimum Cost:  4.5

## Confidence intervals (bootstrap):
##   CI based on normal distribution: 58.76303  -  77.23697
##   CI based on percentiles: 59  -  70
##   Bootstrap resamples: 1000

## Parameters used:
##   Disease prevalence: 0.5
##   Costs (Ctp, Cfp, Ctn, Cfn): 0 1 0 1
##   R: 1
##   Method: empirical
##   Significance Level: 0.05
```

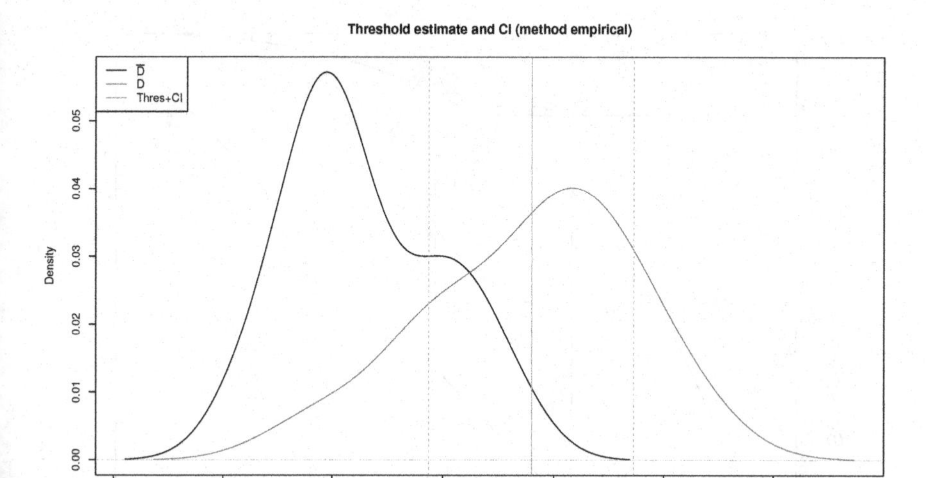

FIGURE 3.9
Illustration of optimal cut-off point selection using the `ThresholdROC` package in `R`.

3.2.5 Sensitivity and Specificity at specific cut-off points

A cut-off point corresponds to a pair of sensitivity and specificity values that characterize the diagnostic marker under study. Confidence intervals for the specificity (or 1-specificity) and sensitivity pair are routinely calculated based on classic binomial distribution formulas [204]. However, when the optimal cut-off point is estimated from the data, rather than considered fixed, the corresponding specificity and sensitivity proportions are correlated and their variability changes accordingly. This correlation needs to be taken into account in order to construct confidence intervals with the correct coverage [16]. McClish (2012) [167] has emphasized the importance of examining the ROC curves of biomarkers in a region around the optimal point.

In order to take into account the correlation between $\hat{\delta}_1 = \frac{c^*-\mu_1}{\sigma_1}$ and $\hat{\delta}_2 = \frac{\mu_2-c^*}{\sigma_2}$, one can construct elliptical confidence regions based on bivariate normality properties. The covariance between $\hat{\delta}_1$ an $\hat{\delta}_2$ can be readily obtained as

$$\begin{aligned} Cov(\hat{\delta}_1, \hat{\delta}_2) \approx & (\frac{\partial\hat{\delta}_2}{\partial\mu_1})(\frac{\partial\hat{\delta}_1}{\partial\mu_1})Var(\hat{\mu}_1) + (\frac{\partial\hat{\delta}_2}{\partial\sigma_1})(\frac{\partial\hat{\delta}_1}{\partial\sigma_1})Var(\hat{\sigma}_1) \\ & + (\frac{\partial\hat{\delta}_2}{\partial\mu_2})(\frac{\partial\hat{\delta}_1}{\partial\mu_2})Var(\hat{\mu}_2) + (\frac{\partial\hat{\delta}_2}{\partial\sigma_2})(\frac{\partial\hat{\delta}_1}{\partial\sigma_2})Var(\hat{\sigma}_2). \end{aligned} \quad (3.28)$$

Let

$$\hat{\mathbf{\Sigma}} = \begin{pmatrix} Var(\hat{\delta}_2) & Cov(\hat{\delta}_2, \hat{\delta}_1) \\ Cov(\hat{\delta}_2, \hat{\delta}_1) & Var(\hat{\delta}_1) \end{pmatrix}.$$

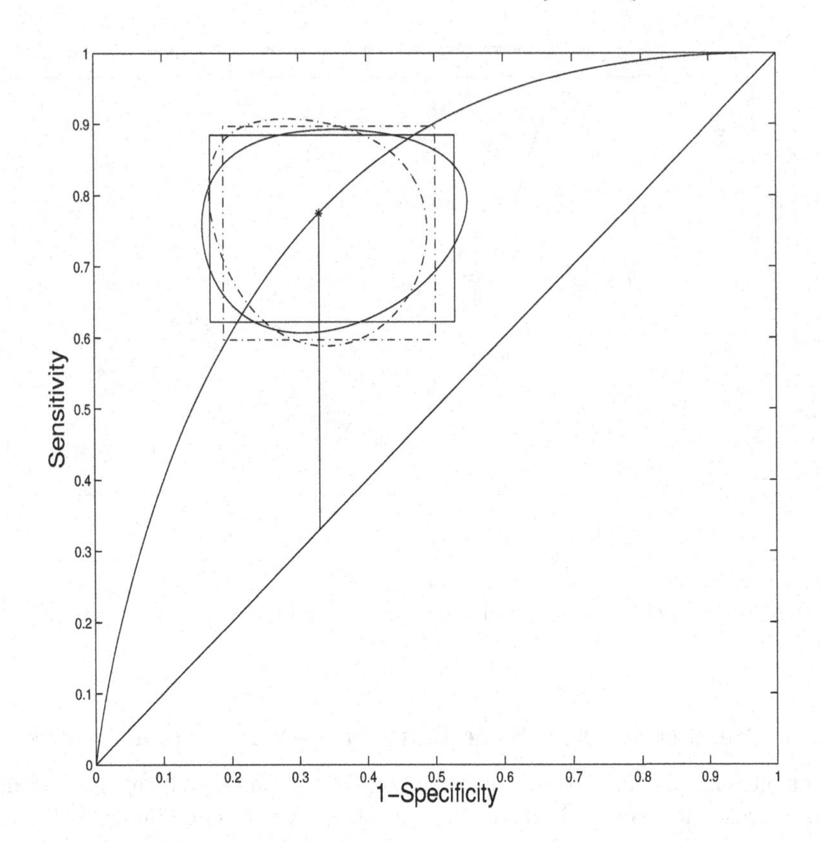

FIGURE 3.10
Delta method (solid lines) and bootstrap (dashed lines) approaches under the binormal model for the construction of confidence regions for the optimal cut-off point [16].

The ellipse defined by $(\mathbf{x}-\mathbf{a})^t\hat{\mathbf{\Sigma}}^{-1}(\mathbf{x}-\mathbf{a}) = q^2$, where $\mathbf{a} = (\hat{\delta}_e, \hat{\delta}_p)$ and q^2 is the 95% percentile of a χ^2_2, is an approximate 95% confidence region for (δ_1, δ_2). Formulas for the partial derivatives that appear in the expressions of $Var(\hat{\delta}_1)$, $Var(\hat{\delta}_2)$, and $Cov(\hat{\delta}_1, \hat{\delta}_2)$ are given in Bantis et al (2014) [16]. The elliptical confidence regions are expected to perform better than the rectangular ones, especially if the correlation between $\hat{\delta}_1$ and $\hat{\delta}_2$ is relatively high. Once we transform back to the ROC space, *i.e.* to the $(1-spec, sens)$ space, we obtain a more irregular shape which represents a 95% confidence region for $(1-spec(c^*), sens(c^*))$.

Alternatively, a standard bootstrap approach or a nonparametric analogue of this procedure can be used as described in Bantis et al. (2014) [16]. `R` and `MATLAB` code for the implementation of the described methods is also provided therein. An illustration is provided in Figure 3.10.

3.3 Exercises

3.1 Estimate the empirical, binormal, and kernel-smoothed ROC curve for the Pancreatic carcinoma data (Section 1.4.3).

3.2 Estimate the AUC and its variance for the Pancreatic carcinoma data using the empirical approach or the binormal assumption.

3.3 Check the null hypothesis: $H_0 : AUC = 0.5$ for the Pancreatic carcinoma data based on resampling methods (bootstrap, permutation methods).

3.4 Estimate the maximum of the Youden index and the respective optimal cut-off point of the ROC curve empirically or under the binormal assumption for the Pancreatic carcinoma data.

3.5 Study the discrepancies between the different methods of obtaining confidence intervals for the AUC under different distributional scenarios for "diseased" vs. "non-diseased".

3.6 For the S-MMSE data consider the PD-MCI vs PD-D patients. Verify the following results: for the empirical approach, the AUC is equal to 0.794 (0.680, 0.908). For the binormal model $\hat{AUC} = 0.794$ (0.661, 0.890). For the kernel-based approach $\hat{AUC} = 0.785$ (0.671, 0.899). The 95% confidence intervals are shown in parentheses. Figure 3.11 depicts the $(1 - spec(c), sens(c))$ empirical pairs along with the binormal (left panel) and the nonparametric kernel (right panel) models for the ROC curve. The AUC was estimated for each case along with 95% confidence intervals. [Tip: The delta method to be used for the construction of confidence intervals under the binormal model, while the bootstrap for the construction of confidence intervals for the kernel-based model. Slight discrepancies for 95% CIs to be expected when the bootstrap is employed. Using `Stata` for the empirical approach, the method by De Long et al. (1988) [64] is implemented through the command `roctab group smmse, graph summary`), where `group` is the binary variable used as reference standard and `smmse` contains the S-MMSE scores].

3.7 For the S-MMSE data consider the PD-MCI vs PD-D patients. Verify that the maximum of the Youden index is 0.445, corresponding to an optimal cut-off point of $c = 24.166$ with $sens(c) = 0.775$ (0.643, 0.874) and $spec(c) = 0.670$ (0.496, 0.813). Marginal 95% confidence intervals for sensitivity and specificity in parentheses are based on the delta method.

3.8 For the S-MMSE data consider the PD-MCI vs PD-D patients. Verify that the approach proposed Metz et al. (1998) [170] for fitting a binormal model with continuous-scaled data results in $\hat{AUC}_L = 0.804$ (0.694, 0.914).

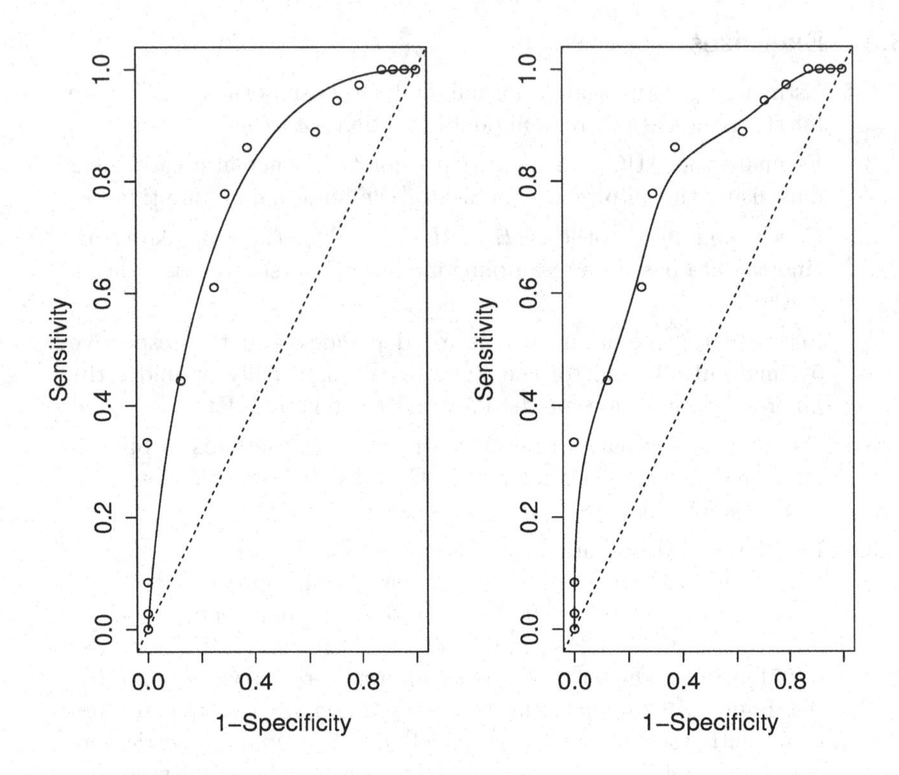

FIGURE 3.11
Left panel: Binormal ROC model for marker S-MMSE (Parkinson disease data). Right panel: Kernel smoothing approach for the same data. Empirical (1-spec, sens) points are provided for reference.

3.9 Study the use of `R` packages `OptimalCutpoints`, `cutpointr`, and `InformationValue` in comparison with results from `ThresholdROC` for the S-MMSE data and PD-MCI vs PD-D patients.

4

Comparing ROC Curves

CONTENTS

4.1 General Considerations 86
4.2 Comparing ROC Curves via their AUC 86
4.2.1 Parametric AUC comparisons 87
4.2.1.1 Ordinal categorical test data 87
4.2.1.2 Normally distributed, continuous test data .. 87
4.2.1.3 Non-normally distributed, continuous test data 89
4.2.1.4 Tests based on the binormal model 91
4.2.2 Nonparametric AUC comparisons 93
4.2.2.1 A general method using U-statistics 93
4.2.2.2 Bootstrap and other alternative nonparametric methods 94
4.3 Comparing ROC Curves via their Youden Index 95
4.3.1 Comparison for normally distributed marker data 96
4.3.2 Comparisons without the normality assumption 98
4.3.3 Nonparametric kernel-based comparisons 98
4.3.4 Omnibus comparisons of ROC curves 100
4.3.4.1 Parametric methods for omnibus ROC curve comparisons 100
4.3.4.2 A nonparametric method for omnibus ROC curve comparisons 103
4.4 AUC-based Testing for Equivalence or Non-inferiority of Diagnostic Tests 104
4.5 Sample Size Considerations 105
4.5.1 Sample size for inference about a single AUC 106
4.5.2 Sample size for comparing two AUCs 106
4.5.3 Choice of metric for ROC comparisons 108
4.6 Exercises 109

DOI: 10.1201/9780429170140-4

4.1 General Considerations

Although an overall comparison of two or more ROC curves can be informative and is often done graphically at the beginning of an analysis, actionable formal comparisons are typically made on the basis of curve summary measures. We introduced several such measures in Section 2.2.3 and discussed statistical methods for their estimation in Chapter 3. This chapter is devoted to the description of the most widely used statistical methods for comparing summaries measures of ROC curves. We focus primarily on the comparison of two curves and indicate how the methodology can be extended to the comparison of more than two curves. Regression analysis of ROC curves is the topic of Chapter 6. At the end of the present chapter, we also discuss study design and sample size considerations for ROC curve comparisons.

The choice of an ROC summary measure for a comparison naturally depends on the scientific or clinical question of interest. When test performance over a range of potential thresholds of test positivity is the main question, as is often the case in diagnostic technology assessment studies, comparisons are made on the basis of the area under the ROC curve (AUC). Other options include the respective maximum of the Youden index (see Section 2.2.3.2) or the length of the ROC curve [89]. When a specific range of thresholds or operating points is of interest, comparisons are made on the basis of the partial area under the ROC curve, the sensitivity at a given value of specificity, or the specificity at a given value of sensitivity. In many situations, several of these measures would be of interest, as they provide complementary information about the test or marker. However, if formal testing of each measure is desired, the analysis would need to address the issue of the multiplicity of inferences.

4.2 Comparing ROC Curves via their AUC

As discussed in the previous chapter (Section 3.2), AUC estimates can be derived using parametric, nonparametric, or bootstrap methods. Because the comparison of AUCs needs to take into consideration if the estimates were obtained on the basis of independent or correlated test (marker) values, the statistical approach needs to account for the nature of the test data, that is, ordinal categorical or continuous and for the *design* of the study. In Section 4.5 we discuss alternative designs and note that designs in which markers are observed on independent samples of participants tend to be less efficient for comparative analyses. More commonly, comparative studies rely on the so-called "paired" designs, in which the markers are assessed on the same set of participants. Naturally, such designs may not always be feasible in practice.

To fix ideas, in a study to compare tests A and B, we assume that, for test A, n_1^A, n_2^A observations are available on participants with and without the target condition, respectively, and, similarly, n_1^B, n_2^B observations are available for test B. The test values for A are denoted by X_{1A}, and X_{2A} and similarly for test B. Test values will be correlated or uncorrelated depending on the particular design. In a paired design, the number of participants with and without the target condition will be the same for A and B. In subsequent discussions of the paired design, we will omit the subscript indicating test and simply denote the sample sizes by n_1, n_2.

4.2.1 Parametric AUC comparisons

4.2.1.1 Ordinal categorical test data

For *ordinal categorical* test data, such as those obtained from the interpretation of diagnostic imaging tests (see the DMIST study case of Section 1.4.5) the area under the ROC curve can be estimated using the original approach of Dorfman and Alf (1969) [69] or using an ordinal regression model as discussed in Section 3.1.1.2. When the curves are estimated on the basis of independent data, the AUC estimates have independently asymptotic normal distributions, which can be used to develop confidence intervals and tests for the difference in AUC. For example, the variance of the difference of AUC estimates would be $\hat{var}(AUC^A - AUC^B) = \hat{var}(AUC_A) + \hat{var}(AUC_B)$ and the estimate of this variance can be used to construct a confidence interval for the difference and corresponding hypothesis tests. When the AUCs are estimated on the basis of correlated test data, the variance of the difference includes also a covariance term.

4.2.1.2 Normally distributed, continuous test data

Wieand et al. (1989) [289] discussed the comparison of AUCs for curves estimated on the basis of *continuous, normally distributed* test data. Specifically, if X_{1A} follows a $N(\mu_{1A}, \sigma_{1A}^2)$ distribution and X_{2A} follows a $N(\mu_{2A}, \sigma_{2A}^2)$ distribution, and $\delta_A = \frac{\mu_{2A} - \mu_{1A}}{\sqrt{\sigma_{2A}^2 + \sigma_{1A}^2}}$ then the area under the ROC curve for test (marker) A is $\Phi(\delta_A)$ and its estimator $\hat{\delta}_A$ is obtained from the corresponding estimates $\hat{\mu}_{1A}, \hat{\mu}_{2A}, \hat{\sigma}_{1A}, \hat{\sigma}_{2A}$. Similar quantities can be derived for marker B and the asymptotic distribution of the statistic $\Delta = \delta_B - \delta_A$ can be obtained from the delta method. This statistic can then be used to test the null hypothesis $H_0 : \delta^A = \delta^B$, which is in turn equivalent to $H_0 : AUC_A = AUC_B$.

For the paired design, if $\sigma_A^2 = \sigma_{1A}^2 + \sigma_{2A}^2$, $C_1 = cov(X_{1A}, X_{1B})$, and $C_2 = cov(X_{2A}, X_{2B})$, then $\sqrt{(n_1 + n_2)} \cdot \Delta$ is asymptotically normal with

$$var(\sqrt{(n_1 + n_2)} \cdot \Delta) = \sigma_{AA} - 2 \cdot \sigma_{AB} + \sigma_{BB},$$

where,

$$\frac{\sigma_{kk}}{n_1+n_2} = \frac{\frac{\sigma_{1k}^2}{n_1}+\frac{\sigma_{2k}^2}{n_2}}{\sigma_k^2} + \frac{\delta_k^2}{2\sigma_k^4}\left(\frac{\sigma_{1k}^4}{n_1-1}+\frac{\sigma_{2k}^4}{n_2-1}\right),$$

$$\frac{\sigma_{AB}}{n_1+n_2} = \frac{\frac{C_1}{n_1}+\frac{C_2}{n_2}}{\sigma_A\sigma_B} + \frac{\delta_A\delta_B}{2(\sigma_A\sigma_B)^2}\left(\frac{C_1^2}{n_1-1}+\frac{C_2^2}{n_2-1}\right).$$

Computations can be performed using R as illustrated below using the LOS data for the comparison of diagnostic markers sTREM-1 and IL-6.

```
wieand.test<-function(x1,y1,x2,y2){
  meanx1<-mean(x1)
  meanx2<-mean(x2)
  stdx1<-sd(x1) ;     stdx2<-sd(x2)
  meany1<-mean(y1)
  meany2<-mean(y2)
  stdy1<-sd(y1)  ;     stdy2<-sd(y2)
  m<-length(x1)  ;     n<-length(y1)

auc.1<-pnorm((meany1-meanx1)/sqrt(stdx1^2+stdy1^2))
auc.2<-pnorm((meany2-meanx2)/sqrt(stdx2^2+stdy2^2))
delta.1<-(meany1-meanx1)/sqrt(stdx1^2+stdy1^2)
delta.2<-(meany2-meanx2)/sqrt(stdx2^2+stdy2^2)
var1w<-var(x1)+var(y1)
var2w<-var(x2)+var(y2)
covxs<-cov(x1,x2)
covys<-cov(y1,y2)

sigma11<-(m+n)*((var(x1)/m+var(y1)/n)/var1w+
0.5*delta.1^2/var1w^2*(var(x1)^2/(m-1)+var(y1)^2/(n-1)))
sigma22<-(m+n)*((var(x2)/m+var(y2)/n)/var2w+
0.5*delta.2^2/var2w^2*(var(x2)^2/(m-1)+var(y2)^2/(n-1)))
sigma12<-(m+n)*((covxs/m+covys/n)/(sqrt(var1w)*sqrt(var2w))+
(0.5*delta.1*delta.2/(var1w*var2w))*(covxs^2/(m-1)
+covys^2/(n-1)))
denomT<-sqrt(sigma11-2*sigma12+sigma22)
wieand.T<-sqrt(m+n)*abs(delta.1-delta.2)/denomT
wieand.p<-2*(1-pnorm(wieand.T))
return(list(auc.1,auc.2,wieand.T,wieand.p)) }

tremdatabasic<-tremdatabasic[-c(47),] #missing value issue
tremx<-tremdatabasic$TREM1[tremdatabasic[,2]==0]
tremy<-tremdatabasic$TREM1[tremdatabasic[,2]==1]
il6x<-tremdatabasic$IL6[tremdatabasic[,2]==0]
il6y<-tremdatabasic$IL6[tremdatabasic[,2]==1]
wieand.test(tremx,tremy,il6x,il6y)
```

```
## [[1]]
## [1] 0.6592511

## [[2]]
## [1] 0.9072123

## [[3]]
## [1] 2.8861

## [[4]]
## [1] 0.003900485
```

Using this procedure, we conclude that IL-6 is a significantly better diagnostic marker than s-TREM1 for the diagnosis of late onset sepsis in neonates ($p = 0.004$). IL-6 results in an AUC of 0.907, while for s-TREM1, $AUC = 0.659$.

4.2.1.3 Non-normally distributed, continuous test data

In practice, the assumption of normality can be rather restrictive and may not be justified by the data at hand, as is the case for the LOS data. In such cases, a power transformation to normality might be preferable. The Box-Cox transformation [36] has often been used for this purpose under the ROC framework [16, 84, 87]. Molodianovitch et al. (2006) [176] have studied the use of the Box-Cox transformation to binormality prior to using the test of Wieand et al. (1989) [289] for AUC comparisons. Through simulations, they conclude that even when the normality assumption does hold for X_{1A}, X_{2A}, and X_{1B}, X_{2B}, their approach has in general higher statistical power than alternatives.

Under the setting in Molodianovitch et al. (2006) [176], two transformation parameters are needed, λ_A and λ_B, one for each biomarker [25,176]. The Box-Cox transformation is defined as $X_{ik}^{(\lambda_k)} = \frac{X_{ik}^{\lambda_k}-1}{\lambda_k}$ for $\lambda_k \neq 0$ and $X_{ik}^{(\lambda_k)} = log(X_{ik})$ otherwise, with $i = 1,2$ and $k \in \{A, B\}$. It is then assumed that the transformed measurements conform to the normality assumption, that is: $X_{ik}^{(\lambda_k)} \sim N(\mu_{ik}^{(\lambda_k)}, {\sigma_{ik}^{(\lambda_k)}}^2)$.

The transformation parameters, along with all underlying means and variances, can be estimated by maximizing the following log-likelihood:

$$\begin{aligned}
&-\frac{n_1}{2}\log(1-\rho_1^2) - \frac{1}{2(1-\rho_1^2)}\sum_{j=1}^{n_1}((\frac{X_{1Aj}^{(\lambda_A)} - \mu_{1A}^{(\lambda_A)}}{\sigma_{1A}^{(\lambda_A)}})^2 \\
&- 2\rho_1(\frac{X_{1Aj}^{(\lambda_A)} - \mu_{1A}^{(\lambda_A)}}{\sigma_{1A}^{(\lambda_A)}})(\frac{X_{1Bj}^{(\lambda_B)} - \mu_{1B}^{(\lambda_B)}}{\sigma_{1B}^{(\lambda_B)}}) + (\frac{X_{1Bj}^{(\lambda_B)} - \mu_{1B}^{(\lambda_B)}}{\sigma_{1B}^{(\lambda_B)}})^2) \\
&+ (\lambda_A - 1)\sum_{j=1}^{n_1}\log(X_{1Aj}^{(\lambda_A)}) + (\lambda_B - 1)\sum_{j=1}^{n_1}\log(X_{1Bj}^{(\lambda_B)})
\end{aligned}$$

$$
\begin{aligned}
&- n_1 \log (2\pi\sigma_{1A}^{(\lambda_A)}\sigma_{1B}^{(\lambda_B)}) - \frac{n_2}{2}\log (1-\rho_2^2) - \frac{1}{2(1-\rho_2^2)}\sum_{l=1}^{n_2}((\frac{X_{2Al}^{(\lambda_A)} - \mu_{2A}^{(\lambda_A)}}{\sigma_{2A}^{(\lambda_A)}})^2 \\
&- 2\rho_2(\frac{X_{2Al}^{(\lambda_A)} - \mu_{2A}^{(\lambda_A)}}{\sigma_{2A}^{(\lambda_A)}})(\frac{X_{2Bl}^{(\lambda_B)} - \mu_{2B}^{(\lambda_B)}}{\sigma_{2B}^{(\lambda_B)}}) + (\frac{X_{2Bl}^{(\lambda_B)} - \mu_{2B}^{(\lambda_B)}}{\sigma_{2B}^{(\lambda_B)}})^2) \\
&+ (\lambda_A - 1)\sum_{l=1}^{n_2}\log (X_{2Al}^{(\lambda_A)}) + (\lambda_B - 1)\sum_{l=1}^{n_2}\log (X_{2Bl}^{(\lambda_B)}) \\
&- n_2 \log (2\pi\sigma_{2A}^{(\lambda_A)}\sigma_{2B}^{(\lambda_B)}),
\end{aligned}
\tag{4.1}
$$

where $\rho_i = corr(X_{iA}^{(\lambda_A)}, X_{iB}^{(\lambda_B)})$, i.e. the correlation coefficient of the transformed measurements between the two markers for each group. We now illustrate the implementation of the Molodianovitch et al. (2006) [176] in R.

```
x1<-tremx
y1<-tremy
x2<-il6x
y2<-il6y
m<-length(x1)
n<-length(y1)

roxlik2<-function(h)
{
  h1<-h[1]  ;   h2<-h[2]
  xh1<-((x1^h1)-1)/h1
  yh1<-((y1^h1)-1)/h1
  xh2<-((x2^h2)-1)/h2
  yh2<-((y2^h2)-1)/h2
  meanxh1<-mean(xh1)
  meanxh2<-mean(xh2)
  stdxh1<-sd(xh1)  ;     stdxh2<-sd(xh2)
  meanyh1<-mean(yh1)
  meanyh2<-mean(yh2)
  stdyh1<-sd(yh1)  ;    stdyh2<-sd(yh2)
  cor1<-cor(xh1,xh2)
  cor2<-cor(yh1,yh2)
  loglik<--(-m/2*log(1-cor1^2)-
   1/(2*(1-cor1^2))*sum((xh1-meanxh1)^2/
     stdxh1^2-2*cor1*((xh1-meanxh1)/stdxh1*(xh2-meanxh2)/stdxh2)+
        (xh2-meanxh2)^2/stdxh2^2)+(h1-1)*sum(log(x1))+
        (h2-1)*sum(log(x2)) -m*log(2*pi*stdxh1*stdxh2)
        -n/2*log(1-cor2^2)-
        1/(2*(1-cor2^2))*sum((yh1-meanyh1)^2/stdyh1^2-
        2*cor2*((yh1-meanyh1)/stdyh1*(yh2-meanyh2)/stdyh2)+
        (yh2-meanyh2)^2/stdyh2^2)+(h1-1)*sum(log(y1))+
            (h2-1)*sum(log(y2))-n*log(2*pi*stdyh1*stdyh2))
  return(loglik)
```

```
}

bclambda<- nlm(roxlik2,c(1,1))

lambda1<-bclambda$estimate[1]
lambda2<-bclambda$estimate[2]

roxcox2 <- function(x1,y1,lambda1,x2,y2,lambda2)
{
  xbc1<-((x1^lambda1)-1)/lambda1
  ybc1<-((y1^lambda1)-1)/lambda1
  xbc2<-((x2^lambda2)-1)/lambda2
  ybc2<-((y2^lambda2)-1)/lambda2
  return(list(xbc1,ybc1, xbc2,ybc2))
}

normlos<-roxcox2(tremx,tremy,lambda1,il6x,il6y,lambda2)

tremxbc<-normlos[[1]]  ;  tremybc<-normlos[[2]]
il6xbc<-normlos[[3]]  ;  il6ybc<-normlos[[4]]

wieand.test(tremxbc,tremybc,il6xbc,il6ybc)
```

```
## [[1]]
## [1] 0.7241175

## [[2]]
## [1] 0.9057213

## [[3]]
## [1] 2.255445

## [[4]]
## [1] 0.02410543
```

After the Box-Cox transformation, the null hypothesis of equality of the corresponding AUCs is still rejected (p=0.024). There is a considerable difference in the AUC estimate for marker sTREM-1. Transformed data conform better to normality assumptions, offering more accurate AUC estimates. The function `comparebcAUC` from the `R` package `rocbc` provides equivalent results.

4.2.1.4 Tests based on the binormal model

The binormal model for ROC analysis was described in the previous chapter (Section 3.1.1.3) Estimation can be implemented using the robust `rocfit`

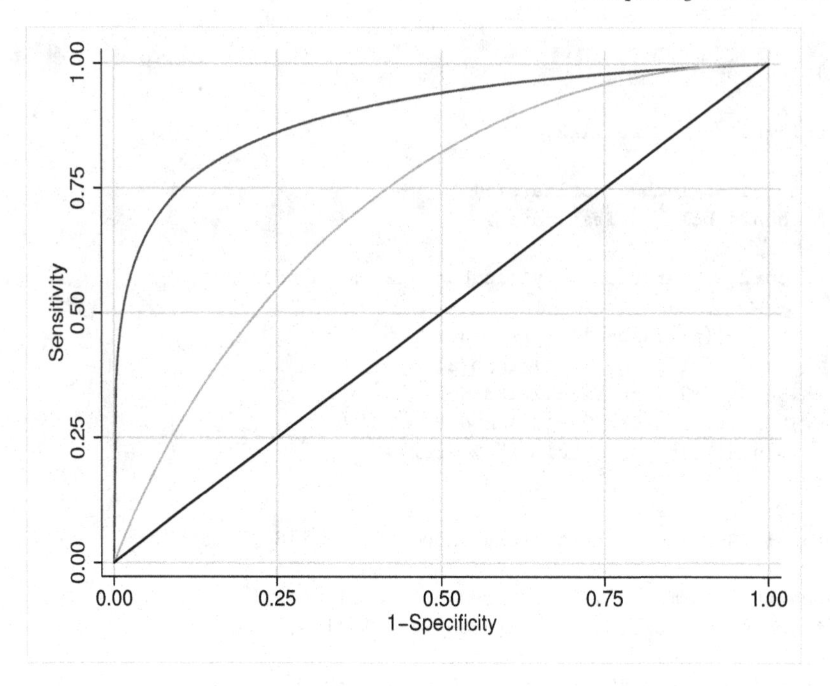

FIGURE 4.1
Illustration of sTREM-1 vs. IL-6 for the prediction of LOS in neonates, binormal ROC estimates are shown.

procedure of Metz et al. (1998) [170]. Comparisons of two AUC estimates from the binormal model are easy to perform using by **Stata** via a simple command:

```
. roccomp D2 TREM1 IL6, graph binormal summary
```

AUC estimates from the binormal model can differ slightly from those obtained via the Box-Cox transformation. For example, the AUC estimate for sTREM-1 under the binormal model is 0.724, (95% CI: 0.582, 0.865) and for IL-6 is 0.899, (95% CI: 0.816, 0.981). Figure 4.1 illustrates the corresponding binormal ROC curves. Their comparison results in $p = 0.033$.

Recall here that the binormal model is known to be quite robust to departures from normality [104] and is also used for analyzing ordinal categorical data.

4.2.2 Nonparametric AUC comparisons

4.2.2.1 A general method using U-statistics

The most widely used nonparametric procedure for AUC comparisons was proposed by DeLong et al. (1988) [64]. The approach uses the theory of U-statistics to derive the asymptotic distribution of the difference of AUC estimates, as described already in Section 3.2.1.1. To fix ideas, in order to evaluate $H_0 : AUC_A = AUC_B$, the test statistic is given by

$$Z_D = \frac{\hat{AUC}_A - \hat{AUC}_B}{\sqrt{\hat{Var}(\hat{AUC}_A) + \hat{Var}(\hat{AUC}_B) - 2 \cdot \hat{Cov}(\hat{AUC}_A, \hat{AUC}_B)}}.$$

The value of the statistic is obtained by using the nonparametric estimates of the areas and their variance, as given in Equations (3.15) and (3.16). The covariance term can be estimated as:

$$\frac{1}{n_1(n_1-1)} \sum_{j=1}^{n_1} [(D_{10}(X_{1j}^A) - \hat{AUC}_A) \cdot (D_{10}(X_{1j}^B) - \hat{AUC}_B)] + \tag{4.2}$$
$$\frac{1}{n_2(n_2-1)} \sum_{i=1}^{n_2} [(D_{01}(X_{2i}^A) - \hat{AUC}_A) \cdot (D_{01}(X_{2i}^B) - \hat{AUC}_B)],$$

where D_{10}, D_{01} are defined according to Equation (3.16). Based on U-statistics properties, $Z_D \sim N(0,1)$.

The development of the method in DeLong et al. (1988) [64] is quite general and covers the general case for the comparison of two or more diagnostic markers according to a contrast of interest. The procedure can be implemented in `R` via the `pROC` package as described below and is also readily offered in `Stata`.

AUC comparisons using a confidence interval approach instead of a testing approach are described in Zou and Yue (2013) [315], while Wieand et al. (1989) [289] describe a method for the comparison of partial AUCs. The latter is asymptotically equivalent to the DeLong et al. (1988) [64] test for the whole AUC.

The markers sTREM-1 and IL-6 are compared in terms of their diagnostic accuracy for the prognosis of LOS in neonates. Figure 4.2 depicts the empirical ROC curves for the two markers using `Stata`:

```
. roccomp D2 TREM1 IL6, graph summary
```

The empirical AUC for sTREM-1 is 0.733 (0.585, 0.882), while for IL-6 it is 0.892 (0.808, 0.976). The test by DeLong et al. (1998) [64] results in $p = 0.053$ The same results can be produced using the `pROC` package by Robin et al. (2011) [221] as follows:

```
library(readxl)
tremdatabasic <- read_excel("Downloads/tremdatabasic.xls")
library(pROC)
Refstd<-tremdatabasic$D2
Zt<-tremdatabasic$TREM1
Zi<-tremdatabasic$IL6
roctrem<-roc(Refstd,Zt)
rocil6<-roc(Refstd,Zi)
roc.test(roctrem,rocil6,method="delong")
```

```
##      DeLong's test for two correlated ROC curves

##    data:  roctrem and rocil6
##    Z = -1.9321, p-value = 0.05335
##    alternative hypothesis: true difference in AUC is not equal to 0
##    95 percent confidence interval:
##    -0.319748331  0.002288013
##    sample estimates:
##    AUC of roc1 AUC of roc2
##    0.7333333   0.8920635
```

4.2.2.2 Bootstrap and other alternative nonparametric methods

Bandos et al. (2005) [14], and Braun and Alonzo (2008) [40] have proposed different permutation tests for the comparison of nonparametric AUCs that result in better small sample performance than the test proposed by DeLong et al. (1988) [64] in many cases. Other resampling approaches that can be used for the nonparametric comparison of two AUCs, such as the bootstrap, have been studied by Moise et al. (1998) [175], Mossman (1995) [180], and Rutter (2000) [228] among others. The `pROC` package [221] in `R` supports the bootstrap comparison of paired AUCs. Specifically, The `"bootstrap"` option for `method` in the `roc.test` function resulted in $p = 0.055$. Based on U-statistics theory [8], it is expected in general that the bootstrap and U-statistics approaches will perform very similarly.

In a non-paired setting, where the measurements for the two markers may arise from different subjects and possibly different sample sizes, the AUC_A and AUC_B are independent and the covariance is zero in all expressions above.

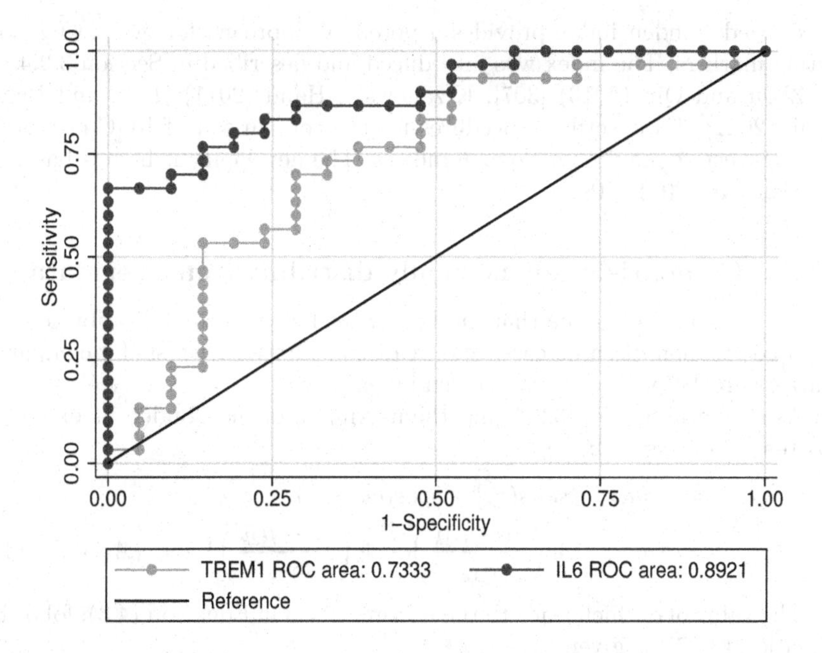

FIGURE 4.2
Illustration of sTREM-1 vs. IL-6 for the prediction of LOS in neonates, empirical ROC estimates are shown. These correspond to the respective binormal ones in Figure 4.1.

Given that there is already provision for the adjustment for ties in the procedure described above, it can be used for ordinal-scaled marker measurements also.

In some cases, the biomarker data are partially paired, that is, for some patients there may exist missing measurements for one of the two markers under study. Zhou and Gatsonis (1996) [312] have expanded the De Long et al. (1988) [64] method for the nonparametric AUC comparison with partially paired data.

4.3 Comparing ROC Curves via their Youden Index

In contrast to the full or partial AUC, which summarize the performance of a marker over a predefined range of values of specificity or sensitivity, the maximized Youden index focuses on an optimised operating point for the marker [302]. In situations when a data driven threshold is desired, the maximized Youden index provides a potential approach for evaluating competing markers. The index was introduced and described in Section 3.2.4.

Zhou and Qin (2013) [307], Krzanowski, Hand (2011) [144], and Bantis et al. (2021) [18] describe procedures for the comparison of ROC curves via their respective maximum Youden indices. The development here is based on Bantis et al. (2021) [18].

4.3.1 Comparison for normally distributed marker data

In this section, we assume that marker values follow normal distributions for diseased and non-diseased cases and we discuss alternative tests for comparing markers on the basis of their Youden index.

As shown in Section 3.2.4 that the maximum of the Youden index can be written as follows [87]:

$$\begin{aligned} J_k &= max_{c_k}\{sens(c_k) + spec(c_k) - 1\} \\ &= max_{c_k}\{\Phi\left(\frac{c_k - \mu_{1k}}{\sigma_{1k}}\right) - \Phi\left(\frac{c_k - \mu_{2k}}{\sigma_{2k}}\right)\}, k \in \{A, B\}. \end{aligned} \tag{4.3}$$

The value of c which leads to the maximization in Equation (4.3), following Equation (3.27), is given by:

$$c_k^* = \frac{\sigma_{1k}^2\mu_{2k} - \sigma_{2k}^2\mu_{1k} - \sigma_{1k}\sigma_{2k}\sqrt{(\mu_{1k} - \mu_{2k})^2 + (\sigma_{1k} - \sigma_{2k}^2)log\frac{\sigma_{1k}^2}{\sigma_{2k}^2}}}{\sigma_{1k}^2 - \sigma_{2k}^2}, \tag{4.4}$$

for $\sigma_{1k} \neq \sigma_{2k}$. The case of equal variances, $\sigma_{1k} = \sigma_{2k}$, yields $c_k^* = (\mu_{1k} + \mu_{2k})/2$.

The corresponding estimator of the maximized Youden index is obtained by using the maximum likelihood estimates of the underlying parameters:

$$\hat{J}_k = \Phi\left(\frac{\hat{c}_k^* - \hat{\mu}_{1k}}{\hat{\sigma}_{1k}}\right) - \Phi\left(\frac{\hat{c}_k^* - \hat{\mu}_{2k}}{\hat{\sigma}_{2k}}\right), k \in \{A, B\}. \tag{4.5}$$

For testing the null hypothesis $H_0 : J_A = J_B$ against $H_a : J_A \neq J_B$, one can use the test statistic:

$$Z = \frac{\hat{J}_B - \hat{J}_A}{\sqrt{Var(\hat{J}_A) + Var(\hat{J}_B) - 2 \cdot Cov(\hat{J}_A, \hat{J}_B)}}, \tag{4.6}$$

which is considered to asymptotically follow a standard normal distribution under the null hypothesis. Z can straightforwardly be adapted to examine one-sided alternatives.

By applying the delta method, we obtain the following approximation of the variance of the estimated index:

$$Var\left(\hat{J}_k\right) \approx \left(\frac{\partial \hat{J}_k}{\partial \mu_{1k}}, \frac{\partial \hat{J}_k}{\partial \sigma_{1k}}, \frac{\partial \hat{J}_k}{\partial \mu_{2k}}, \frac{\partial \hat{J}_k}{\partial \sigma_{2k}}\right) \hat{\Sigma}_i \left(\frac{\partial \hat{J}_k}{\partial \mu_{1k}}, \frac{\partial \hat{J}_k}{\partial \sigma_{1k}}, \frac{\partial \hat{J}_k}{\partial \mu_{2k}}, \frac{\partial \hat{J}_k}{\partial \sigma_{2k}}\right)', \tag{4.7}$$

where $k \in \{A, B\}$ and $\hat{\Sigma}_k$ is the estimated covariance matrix that refers to the vector of parameters $(\mu_{1k}, \sigma_{1k}, \mu_{2k}, \sigma_{2k})$.

The corresponding approximation for the covariance term in Equation (4.6) is given by:

$$Cov(\hat{J}_A, \hat{J}_B) \approx \left(\frac{\partial \hat{J}_A}{\partial \mu_{1A}}, \frac{\partial \hat{J}_A}{\partial \sigma_{1A}}, 0, 0, \frac{\partial \hat{J}_A}{\partial \mu_{2A}}, \frac{\partial \hat{J}_A}{\partial \sigma_{2A}}, 0, 0 \right) \hat{\Sigma}^* \left(0, 0, \frac{\partial \hat{J}_B}{\partial \mu_{1B}}, \frac{\partial \hat{J}_B}{\partial \sigma_{1B}}, 0, 0 \frac{\partial \hat{J}_B}{\partial \mu_{2B}}, \frac{\partial \hat{J}_B}{\partial \sigma_{2B}} \right)' . \quad (4.8)$$

The partial derivatives involved in Equations (4.7) and (4.8) and the form of $\hat{\Sigma}_i$ are provided in Schisterman and Perkins (2007) [235]. Derivation of the matrix $\hat{\Sigma}^*$ involved in Equation (4.8) is given in Bantis and Feng (2016) [25]. Specifically, $\hat{\Sigma}^*$ is obtained by inverting the corresponding estimated Fisher information matrix (see Web Appendix in Bantis et al. (2021) [18]). The information matrix is estimated by substituting the maximum likelihood estimates of the underlying parameters.

An alternative test statistic can be obtained by using a transformation of the Youden index estimate as described by Bantis et al. (2019) [17]. The resulting statistic is given by:

$$Z^* = \frac{\hat{J}_{TB} - \hat{J}_{TA}}{\sqrt{Var(\hat{J}_{TA}) + Var(\hat{J}_{TB}) - 2 \cdot Cov(\hat{J}_{TA}, \hat{J}_{TB})}}, \quad (4.9)$$

where $\hat{J}_{Tk} = log\frac{0.5(\hat{J}_k+1)}{1-0.5(\hat{J}_k+1)}$, $k \in \{A, B\}$ with

$$Var(\hat{J}_{Tk}) \approx \frac{4}{(\hat{J}_k^2 - 1)^2} \times Var(\hat{J}_k) \quad (4.10)$$

and

$$Cov(\hat{J}_{TA}, \hat{J}_{TB}) \approx \frac{16}{(\hat{J}_B^2 - 1)^2(\hat{J}_A^2 - 1)^2} \times Cov(\hat{J}_A, \hat{J}_B).$$

Under the null hypothesis, Z^* also follows an asymptotically standard normal distribution.

Alternative transformations include $\hat{J}_T = \Phi^{-1}(\hat{J})$, as well as $\hat{J}_T = logit(\hat{J})$. The resulting statistics are very similar, as discussed in Bantis et al. (2021) [18].

The corresponding $1 - \alpha$ confidence intervals for the difference of the maximized Youden indices are

$$\left(\hat{dJ} - Z_{1-\frac{\alpha}{2}} \times \sqrt{Var\left(\hat{dJ}\right)}, \hat{dJ} + Z_{1-\frac{\alpha}{2}} \times \sqrt{Var\left(\hat{dJ}\right)} \right), \quad (4.11)$$

where $\hat{dJ} = \hat{J}_B - \hat{J}_A$ and $Z_{1-\frac{\alpha}{2}}$ is the α level's Z-score for a two-tailed test. The variance term $Var(\hat{dJ})$ is calculated by using $Var(\hat{dJ}) = Var(\hat{J}_{TA}) + Var(\hat{J}_{TB}) - 2 \cdot Cov(\hat{J}_{TA}, \hat{J}_{TB})$.

4.3.2 Comparisons without the normality assumption

For non-normally distributed marker data, the Box-Cox transformation, as described in Section 4.2.1, can be readily used for the comparison of the two maximized Youden indices of competing biomarkers. Details are provided in Bantis et al. (2021) [18]. The R package rocbc was specifically built for the implementation of Box-Cox transformation methods in ROC curve analysis. An example with simulated data follows for the comparison of two maximized Youden indices.

```
library(calibrate)
library(rocbc)
set.seed(123)
nx = 100; ny = 100
Sx = matrix(c(1, 0.5, 0.5, 1), nrow = 2, ncol = 2)
mux= c(X = 10, Y = 12)
X=rmvnorm(nx, mean = mux, sigma = Sx)

Sy = matrix(c(1.1, 0.6, 0.6, 1.1), nrow = 2, ncol = 2)
muy = c(X = 11, Y = 13.7)
Y=rmvnorm(ny, mean = muy, sigma = Sy)

dx=zeros(nx,1); dy=ones(ny,1)
markers=rbind(X,Y);
markerA=markers[,1] ; markerB=markers[,2]
D=c(rbind(dx,dy))

# markerA: measurements for marker A for all individuals.
# markerB: measurements for marker B for all individuals.
# D: status (0 for non-diseased, 1 for diseased).

out=comparebcJ(markerA, markerB , D , plots=on); out$resultstable
```

We obtain a table with estimates of J for markers A, B ($J_A = 0.451$, $J_B = 0.619$), the corresponding $p = 0.002$ and 95% confidence intervals for the difference between the two Youden indices.

4.3.3 Nonparametric kernel-based comparisons

Nonparametric kernel-based methods for estimating an ROC curve were discussed in Section 3.1.3.1 of the book. Such methods can also be used to compare curves if transformation to normality cannot be obtained. Naturally, such methods need to take into account the correlation induced by a paired study design.

In this section we discuss the use of product-based bivariate kernel density estimation to compare two correlated Youden indices. For the non-diseased group, the estimator is defined as:

$$\hat{f}_1(x_{1A}, x_{1B}) = \frac{1}{n_1 h_{1A} h_{1B}} \sum_{i=1}^{n_1} K\left(\frac{x_{1A} - X_{1Aj}}{h_{1A}}\right) K\left(\frac{x_{1B} - X_{1Bj}}{h_{1B}}\right), \quad (4.12)$$

The estimator $\hat{f}_2(x_{2A}, x_{2B})$ for the diseased group is defined similarly. The normal kernel $K(t) = \frac{1}{\sqrt{2\pi}} e^{-\frac{t^2}{2}}$ can be considered. The bandwidths for the non-diseased individuals are denoted by h_{1A} and h_{1B}, while h_{2A} and h_{2B} are the corresponding bandwidths for the diseased individuals.

For normal kernels, Scott (1992) [238] presents bandwidths that are optimal in terms of the asymptotic integrated mean squared error (AMISE). These are of the form

$$h_{1A} = std(X_{1A})(1 - Corr(X_{1A}, X_{1B})^2)^{5/12}(1 + Corr(X_{1A}, X_{1B})^2/2)^{-1/6} n_1^{-1/6},$$

where $std(X_{1A})$ is the standard deviation for the X_{1A} measurements and $Corr(X_{1A}, X_{1B})$ is the Pearson correlation between the X_{1A} and X_{1B} samples, while n_1 is the sample size for the non-diseased subjects. Plug-in estimates can be directly used to calculate the corresponding bandwidths. The expressions are analogous for the bandwidths h_{1B}, h_{2A}, h_{2B}.

The marginal non-diseased-related cumulative distribution function (cdf) estimate of marker A is denoted as $\hat{F}_{1A}$ and can be obtained by numerical integration. Similarly, we obtain all remaining estimated marginal cdfs $\hat{F}_{1B}$, $\hat{F}_{2A}$ and $\hat{F}_{2B}$. We can obtain the kernel-based ROC estimator for marker A, $\hat{ROC}_A$, by relying on $\hat{F}_{1A}$ and $\hat{F}_{2A}$. Similarly for $\hat{ROC}_B$, we note that the kernel-based estimator of the ROC is a continuous function with respect to t. The corresponding maximized Youden indices can be obtained by numerical optimization performed separately for each of the two estimated ROC curves, $\hat{ROC}_A$ and $\hat{ROC}_B$. We denote these estimators by $\hat{J}_i^{(K)}$, $i \in \{A, B\}$.

To assess whether there is a statistically significant difference between the two maximized Youden indices, we employ the following bootstrap-based algorithm.

- Step 1: Draw paired bootstrap samples of size n_1 and n_2 with replacement from (X_{1A}, X_{2A}) and (X_{1B}, X_{2B}), respectively. These are the current bootstrap samples.

- Step 2: Using the current bootstrap samples obtain the kernel-based $\hat{ROC}_A$ and numerically derive the maximized Youden index. Denote this with $\hat{J}_{A(m)}^{(K)}$ for the current m^{th} bootstrap sample. Work similarly for biomarker B and obtain $\hat{J}_{B(m)}^{(K)}$.

- Step 3: Repeat Steps 1 and 2 M times and derive the bootstrap-based estimates of the variances of $\hat{J}_i^{(K)}$ by calculating $Var\left(\hat{J}_i^{(K)}\right) = \frac{1}{M-1} \sum_{m=1}^{M} \left(\hat{J}_{i(m)}^{(K)} - \bar{\hat{J}}_i^{(K)}\right)^2$, where $\bar{\hat{J}}_i^{(K)}$ is the mean of the M estimates

$\hat{J}_{i(m)}^{(K)}$ for $i \in \{A, B\}$. The corresponding covariances are calculated accordingly based on the M bootstrap samples.

After deriving the variances and covariances mentioned in Step 3, the construction of confidence intervals of the actual difference between the two maximized Youden indices are straightforward and can be derived utilizing Formula (4.11). If the confidence interval does not include zero, the maximized Youden indices will differ significantly. Namely, in this context, the confidence interval corresponds to testing the null hypothesis $H_0 : J_A = J_B$ which is equivalent to evaluating $H_0 : J_A - J_B = 0$ at a given nominal level.

Alternatively, one can also use one of the previously described logit or probit transformations instead of working directly with the maximized Youden indices. Working with a transformation is helpful since the corresponding confidence interval (after back-transforming its endpoints) will not "bleed" out of the domain of the difference of the two maximized Youden indices. In addition, these transformations have been shown to perform well in terms of width and coverage [18].

4.3.4 Omnibus comparisons of ROC curves

A graphical comparison of ROC curves is typically the first step in a data analysis. For theoretical completeness, we discuss here omnibus test procedures for comparing two curves. Such tests may be considered in situations where summary indices, such as J and AUC, may not seem representative or relevant to the particular marker comparison. binormal model-based comparisons are reasonable for ordinal-scaled biomarkers which suffer from large numbers of ties between measurements.

4.3.4.1 Parametric methods for omnibus ROC curve comparisons

Under the binormal assumption, one can test for the equality of two ROC curves via the equality of their corresponding binormal model parameters as initially proposed by Metz, Kronman (1980) [171], and Metz et al. (1984) [173]. A chi-squared test to assess the null hypothesis $H_0 : a_A = a_B$ `AND` $b_A = b_B$, against the alternative with a logical `NAND` instead of an `AND` operator (that is, "not equal" for any or both of the equalities under H_0), is given by,

$$(\hat{a}_A - \hat{a}_B,\ \hat{b}_A - \hat{b}_B) \cdot \Sigma^{-1} \cdot (\hat{a}_A - \hat{a}_B,\ \hat{b}_A - \hat{b}_B)^t \sim \chi_2^2, \tag{4.13}$$

where Σ is the variance-covariance matrix for $(\hat{a}_A - \hat{a}_B,\ \hat{b}_A - \hat{b}_B)$. An illustration of this procedure where a delta method approximation is given for Σ through symbolic programming in `R` follows.

```
mecro.ROC<-function(x1A,x2A,x1B,x2B){

mu1A<-mean(x1A) ; mu2A<-mean(x2A)
si1A<-sd(x1A) ; si2A<-sd(x2A)
mu1B<-mean(x1B) ; mu2B<-mean(x2B)
si1B<-sd(x1B) ; si2B<-sd(x2B)
n1<-length(x1A) ; n2<-length(x2A)

#auc<-pnorm((mu2-mu1)/sqrt(si1^2+si2^2))
alphad<-expression((m2A-m1A)/s2A-((m2B-m1B)/s2B))
betad<-expression(s1A/s2A-(s1B/s2B))

alphm1A<-D(alphad,"m1A")
alphAm1<-eval(alphm1A, list(m1A=mu1A, m2A=mu2A, m1B=mu1B,
m2B=mu2B, s2A=si2A, s2B=si2B))
alphm2A<-D(alphad,"m2A")
alphAm2<-eval(alphm2A, list(m1A=mu1A, m2A=mu2A, m1B=mu1B,
m2B=mu2B, s2A=si2A, s2B=si2B))
alphm1B<-D(alphad,"m1B")
alphBm1<-eval(alphm1B, list(m1A=mu1A, m2A=mu2A, m1B=mu1B,
m2B=mu2B, s2A=si2A, s2B=si2B))
alphm2B<-D(alphad,"m2B")
alphBm2<-eval(alphm2B, list(m1A=mu1A, m2A=mu2A, m1B=mu1B,
m2B=mu2B, s2A=si2A, s2B=si2B))
alphs2A<-D(alphad,"s2A")
alphAs2<-eval(alphs2A, list(m1A=mu1A, m2A=mu2A, m1B=mu1B,
m2B=mu2B, s2A=si2A, s2B=si2B))
alphs2B<-D(alphad,"s2B")
alphBs2<-eval(alphs2B, list(m1A=mu1A, m2A=mu2A, m1B=mu1B,
m2B=mu2B, s2A=si2A, s2B=si2B))

bets1A<-D(betad,"s1A")
betAs1<-eval(bets1A, list(s1A=si1A, s1B=si1B,
s2A=si2A, s2B=si2B))
bets2A<-D(betad,"s2A")
betAs2<-eval(bets2A, list(s1A=si1A, s1B=si1B,
s2A=si2A, s2B=si2B))
bets1B<-D(betad,"s1B")
betBs1<-eval(bets1B, list(s1A=si1A, s1B=si1B,
s2A=si2A, s2B=si2B))
bets2B<-D(betad,"s2B")
betBs2<-eval(bets2B, list(s1A=si1A, s1B=si1B,
s2A=si2A, s2B=si2B))

varad<-alphAm1^2*(si1A^2/n1)+alphAm2^2*(si2A^2/n2)
+alphBm1^2*(si1B^2/n1)+alphBm2^2*(si2B^2/n2)
+alphAs2^2*(si2A^2/(2*(n2-1)))
```

```
+alphBs2^2*(si2B^2/(2*(n2-1)))
varbd<-betAs1^2*(si1A^2/(2*(n1-1)))
+betAs2^2*(si2A^2/(2*(n2-1)))
+betBs1^2*(si1B^2/(2*(n1-1)))
+betBs2^2*(si2B^2/(2*(n2-1)))
covabd<-alphAs2*betAs2*(si2A^2/(2*(n2-1)))
+alphBs2*betBs2*(si2B^2/(2*(n2-1)))

testx2<-t(c((mu2A-mu1A)/si2A-((mu2B-mu1B)/si2B),si1A/si2A
-(si1B/si2B)))%*%solve(matrix(c(varad,covabd,covabd,varbd),2,2))
%*%c((mu2A-mu1A)/si2A-((mu2B-mu1B)/si2B),si1A/si2A
-(si1B/si2B))
### uses function aucsi from Section 3.2.1.2
return(list(aucsi(x1A,x2A), aucsi(x1B,x2B), testx2,
1-pchisq(testx2,2)))
}


tremdata<-read.csv(file.choose()) #tremdatabasic.csv
tremdata<-tremdata[-47,]
trem1x1A<-tremdata[,3][tremdata[,2]==0]
trem1x2A<-tremdata[,3][tremdata[,2]==1]
il6x1B<-tremdata[,4][tremdata[,2]==0]
il6x2B<-tremdata[,4][tremdata[,2]==1]
x1A<-trem1x1A
x2A<-trem1x2A
x1B<-il6x1B
x2B<-il6x2B


mecro.ROC(x1A,x2A,x1B,x2B)
```

```
## [[1]]
## [[1]][[1]]
## [1] 0.6592511
##
## [[1]][[2]]
## [1] 0.5066874

## [[1]][[3]]
## [1] 0.7893237

## [[2]]
## [[2]][[1]]
## [1] 0.9072123
```

```
##   [[2]][[2]]
##   [1] 0.7998431

##   [[2]][[3]]
##   [1] 0.9645801

##   [[3]]
##              [,1]
##   [1,] 17.79341

##   [[4]]
##              [,1]
##   [1,] 0.0001368389
```

Applying the binormal model directly and using Equation (4.13) for the direct comparison of the ROC curves for the LOS data results in a highly significant result with $X_2^2 = 17.793$, $p < 0.001$. The two ROC curves differ significantly in terms of shapes of their binormal estimates. Notice that under the direct application of the binormal model AUC for sTREM-1 is 0.659 (0.507, 0.789), while for IL-6 it is 0.907 (0.800, 0.965).

4.3.4.2 A nonparametric method for omnibus ROC curve comparisons

Venkatraman and Begg (1996) [274] proposed a nonparametric approach for the comparison of entire empirical ROC curves. The approach uses a permutation testing procedure with a summary statistic based on empirical quantiles (rank statistics). The authors provide an example of using their method and claim that the power of the procedure is comparable to the power of the DeLong test when for alternatives in which one ROC curve completely dominates the other and is better for alternatives in which the two ROC curves cross. The procedure is implemented in the `pROC` package.

```
library(readxl)
tremdatabasic <- read_excel("Downloads/tremdatabasic.xls")
library(pROC)
Refstd<-tremdatabasic$D2
Zt<-tremdatabasic$TREM1
Zi<-tremdatabasic$IL6
roctrem<-roc(Refstd,Zt)
rocil6<-roc(Refstd,Zi)

set.seed(2022)
roc.test(roctrem,rocil6,method="venkatraman")
```

```
## |==================================================================| 100%

## Venkatraman's test for two paired ROC curves

## data:  roctrem and rocil6
## E = 200, boot.n = 2000, p-value = 0.078
## alternative hypothesis: true difference in AUC is not equal to 0
```

We get $p = 0.078$ and draw similar conclusions with the DeLong et al. (1988) [64] approach.

Basic methods for paired ROC curve comparison

1. AUC-based, nonparametric: DeLong et al. (1988) [64].
2. AUC-based, parametric, binormal: Wieand et al. (1989) [289].
3. AUC-based, parametric, binormal: Metz et al. (1998) [170].
4. J-based, parametric, binormal: Bantis et al. (2021) [18].
5. J-based, nonparametric: Bantis et al. (2021) [18].
6. Comparison at given *sens* or *spec* level: Bantis and Feng (2016) [25].
7. Direct ROC-based, nonparametric: Venkatraman and Begg (1996) [274].
8. Direct ROC-based, parametric, binormal: Metz et al. (1984) [173].

- Option of using the Box-Cox transformation prior to the assumption of normality and the binormal model for continuous-scaled biomarker measurements.
- Methods 3. and 8 recommended for ordinal-scaled biomarker measurements.

4.4 AUC-based Testing for Equivalence or Non-inferiority of Diagnostic Tests

The assessment of equivalence of therapeutic interventions has received extensive attention in the clinical trials literature [59, 288]. The approaches used to compare therapies can be readily translated to the comparison of diagnostic modalities [196]. Briefly, if θ_A, θ_B represent measures of diagnostic performance of two modalities, such as imaging modalities or biomarkers, equivalence is typically defined as $|\theta_A - \theta_B| < \delta$ where δ is the so-called *margin of equivalence* and is chosen on biomedical subject matter and cost considerations. This formulation of equivalence implies that the two measures of performance differ by at most δ units. Several other versions of equivalence have been considered in the literature, including versions that compare the two measures using metrics other than the difference, such as ratios. Of particular importance is the notion of *non-inferiority.* If marker B is considered the current standard, the non-inferiority of marker A in comparison with marker B is defined as $\theta_A > \theta_B - \delta$, where δ is a non-negative *non-inferiority margin.* In other words, marker A will be declared non-inferior to the standard marker by margin δ of its diagnostic performance if at most δ units below the performance of the standard.

A general approach to assessing non-inferiority or equivalence was proposed by Blackwelder (1982) [33]. To assess non-inferiority, this approach sets the null hypothesis to represent that non-inferiority is *not* satisfied and the alternative hypothesis to represent that non-inferiority *is* satisfied. Formally, $H_0 : \theta_A \leq \theta_B - \delta$ and $H_a : \theta_A > \theta_B - \delta$. If the test rejects H_0, that is, the upper confidence interval for $\theta_A - \theta_B$ is completely above $-\delta$, the conclusion favors the non-inferiority of marker A in comparison with the standard marker B, with non-inferiority margin equal to δ. The testing of the equivalence hypothesis is done similarly.

Alternative procedures for testing for equivalence and/or non-inferiority in the ROC context, not necessarily restricted to the whole AUC, are also described in Li et al. (2008) [148], Liu et al. (2006) [153], Lu et al. (2003) [158], and Obuchowski (2001) [198].

4.5 Sample Size Considerations

The derivation of sample sizes needed for ROC analysis naturally depends on the ROC index of primary interest and the specific hypotheses under consideration. In this section, we survey methods for estimating sample sizes needed to estimate and compare AUCs. In particular, we discuss sample size considerations for the estimation of the AUC of a single curve and of the difference of AUCs of two curves, possibly using correlated observations as is the case in a paired design. For a detailed discussion of design considerations for diagnostic markers, the reader can consult the comprehensive account provided in Chapter 6 of Zhou et al. (2011) [314].

4.5.1 Sample size for inference about a single AUC

As discussed in Section 3.2.1.1, the commonly used nonparametric estimator of the AUC in Equation (3.15) is equivalent to the Wilcoxon–Mann–Whitney statistic. The general formula for the variance of this estimator in Equation (3.18) is somewhat complex. Recall that, when there are no "ties" in the marker data the variance is given by

$$Var(\hat{AUC}) = \frac{1}{n_1 n_2}(AUC(1-AUC) + (n_1-1)(Q_1 - AUC^2) + (n_2-1)(Q_2 - AUC^2)), \quad (4.14)$$

and that Q_1 and Q_2 are estimated by: $\hat{Q}_1 = \frac{AUC}{2-AUC}$ and $\hat{Q}_2 = \frac{2AUC^2}{1+AUC}$. The reader may note that in this formulation, the estimation of the variance requires only the two sample sizes and the postulated AUC value.

The variance formula in (4.14) with the above approximations of Q_1 and Q_2 can be used to derive the sample sizes of diseased and non-diseased subjects needed to achieve a desired length for the confidence interval of an AUC or desired power for a test of a simple null hypothesis about the AUC value. Simulation studies have shown that the approximation of Q_1 and Q_2 under the exponential distribution assumption works reasonably well for markers taking continuous values. For markers taking discrete values, the following approximation, based on the binormal model, has better performance [197]:

$$Var(\hat{AUC}) = 0.0099 \cdot e^{A^2/2}(\frac{5A^2+8}{n_1} + \frac{A^2+8}{n_2}),$$

where $A = 1.414 \cdot \Phi^{-1}(AUC))$ and Φ denotes the standard normal cumulative distribution function.

4.5.2 Sample size for comparing two AUCs

As noted in Section 4.2.2, a test statistic for comparing two areas under the curve has the general form

$$Z_D = \frac{\hat{AUC}_A - \hat{AUC}_B}{\sqrt{\hat{Var}(\hat{AUC}_A) + \hat{Var}(\hat{AUC}_B) - 2 \cdot \hat{Cov}(\hat{AUC}_A, \hat{AUC}_B)}}. \quad (4.15)$$

In order to derive the required sample size for estimation or testing, the analyst would need to use estimates of the variance and covariance terms in this expression. Approximations for the variance of estimates of single curves were discussed in the previous section. An approximation for the covariance term is somewhat more involved to derive.

For the common situation of comparing AUC estimates derived from a paired design, Obuchowski and McClish (1997) [200] proposed the following formula, which is based on a bivariate binormal model for the joint distribution of the marker data:

$$\hat{Cov}(\hat{AUC}_A, \hat{AUC}_B)) = \frac{e^{-(a_1^2+a_2^2)/4}}{12.554}(r_1 + \frac{r_2}{c} + r_1^2 a_1 \frac{a_2}{2}) + \frac{e^{-(a_1^2+a_2^2)/4}}{50.2655}\frac{a_1 a_2 r_2^2 + c r_1^2}{2c},$$

where, $c = n_2/n_1$ is the ratio of sample sizes of nondiseased to diseased subjects, a_1 is the intercept term in the binormal model for area A and a_2 is the corresponding term for area B, r_1 is the correlation in the bivariate binormal model for diseased subjects, and r_2 is the correlation in the bivariate binormal model for non-diseased subjects.

The selection of values for the parameters in Equation (4.15) can require a fair amount of detail that is not necessarily available at the design stage of a study. An alternative approach was proposed by Blume (2009) [35], who worked with the Birnbaum and Klose (1957) [32] bounds on the variance of the usual non-parametric estimate of the AUC and derived general bounds on the variance of the difference between two AUC estimates. These bounds can be used to derive a maximum sample size that is not dependent on the distribution of marker values.

The `pROC` package in `R` implements the procedures described in Obuchowski and McClish (1997) [200] for AUC-based biomarker comparison in a paired setting.

Consider the brucellosis study data described in Section 1.4.1. We will be using the data from this study to help us design a new one that will be powered enough to find a significant difference between markers CD3 and CD4. Notice here that, based on the data at hand, CD3 and CD4 do not differ significantly at the $\alpha = 5\%$ level. This is easy to verify by running the following line of code in `Stata` after importing the data:

```
. roccomp d2 cd4_pha cd3_pha, graph summary
```

The resulting chi-squared statistic with one degree of freedom is equal to 2.56, corresponding to $p = 0.110$. The researchers would like to demonstrate that CD4 is a better biomarker than CD3 in detecting disease. Looking for 80% power at level $\alpha = 5\%$, the following code in `R` provides the sample size needed.

```
library(pROC)
ob.params <- list(A1=1.07, B1=0.68, A2=1.768, B2=0.687, rn=-0.107
, ra=0.597, delta=0.107)

power.roc.test(ob.params, power=0.8, sig.level=0.05, alternative="o")
```

```
##      Two ROC curves power calculation

##          ncases = 83.71559
##       ncontrols = 83.71559
##       sig.level = 0.05
##           power = 0.8
```

We conclude that 84 subjects per group would be needed (controls vs cases) in order to be able to reject the null hypothesis of equality of the corresponding AUCs for CD3 and CD4 versus the one-sided alternative: $AUC_{CD4} > AUC_{CD3}$ with power equal to 80%. This derivation was based on the binormal assumption and the corresponding estimated parameters from the data at hand were directly plugged into the relevant package function. In practice, one may aim for a somewhat larger sample size, e.g. an extra 10%, in order to take dropouts into account. The target sample size will be affected by the nature of the study, which may in turn affect the number of expected dropouts.

4.5.3 Choice of metric for ROC comparisons

The choice of an ROC summary measure for a comparison naturally depends on the scientific or clinical question of interest. When test performance over a range of potential thresholds of test positivity is the main question, as is often the case in diagnostic technology assessment studies, comparisons are made on the basis of the area under the ROC curve (AUC). Other options include the respective maximum of the Youden index (see Section 2.2.3.2) or the length of the ROC curve [20,89]. When a specific range of thresholds or operating points is of interest, comparisons are made on the basis of the partial area under the ROC curve [256], the sensitivity at a given value of specificity, or the specificity at a given value of sensitivity. In many situations, several of these measures would be of interest, as they provide complementary information about the test or marker. However, if formal testing of each measure is desired, the analysis would need to address the issue of the multiplicity of inferences.

The choice of using AUC or J for ROC curve comparison can also be related to the stage of development of the biomarkers under study. For biomarkers at the early stage of development, e.g. prior to their large-scale use in clinical practice, the AUC might be a more appropriate measure since its calculation is based on the whole ROC curve, before an optimal decision threshold has been defined. However, J-based comparisons can be more relevant when the biomarkers under consideration are widely used in practice and an optimal cut-off point has already been defined for each. In any case, one must take into account the applied framework under which the biomarker comparison takes place in order to employ the most appropriate procedure.

4.6 Exercises

4.1 Estimate differences using the `rocbc` package for the LOS data based on the code illustration of Section 4.3.1.

4.2 Assume binormality after applying a Box-Cox transformation and use the `roc.test` function of the `pROC` package in `R` with the "bootstrap" option for the LOS data. Are results comparable with those in Section 4.2.1.4?

4.3 Apply the Metz-Kronman test after a Box-Cox transformation and compare with results of Section 4.3.4.1.

4.4 Compare the procedure described in Section 4.2.1.3 with the results of the function `comparebcAUC` from package `rocbc` using the LOS data.

4.5 A visual representation of different ROC curve estimates and corresponding Youden index-based optimal cut-off/operating points for the pancreatic cancer data (Section 1.4.3) is given in Figure 4.3.

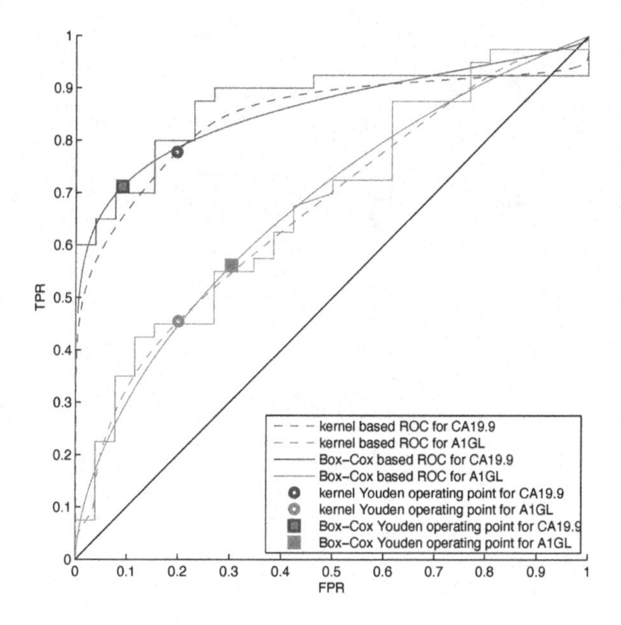

FIGURE 4.3
ROC curves for CA19-9 and A1GL for the pancreatic cancer data. Along with the Box-Cox and kernel-based ROC curves for both markers. The empirical ROC estimates are also presented.

The discrimination capacity of selected markers for cancer patients vs subjects with pancreatitis is assessed and compared. Verify that AUC-based and J-based methods all produce statistically significant differences between the corresponding indices for the two markers under consideration.

5

The ROC Surface and k-class Classification for $k > 2$

CONTENTS

5.1 The ROC Surface for Ordered Three-class Classification 112
  5.1.1 The three-class model 112
  5.1.2 ROC surface modelling 114
    5.1.2.1 Empirical and general nonparametric estimation 114
    5.1.2.2 Parametric estimation, the trinormal model . 115
5.2 The Volume Under the ROC Surface (VUS) and its Estimation 118
5.3 Hypothesis Testing for VUS 119
  5.3.1 Hypothesis testing for a single VUS 119
  5.3.2 Comparison of diagnostic markers via their VUS estimates 121
5.4 Hypothesis Testing for the Entire ROC Surface 122
  5.4.1 Comparing two markers 122
  5.4.2 Box-Cox transformation when comparing two markers . 125
  5.4.3 Special case: Assessment of a single marker 126
5.5 The ROC Umbrella, Different Order Restrictions 127
5.6 ROC Hypersurfaces, Multiple-class Classification 129
5.7 Generalized Youden Index, Cut-off Point Selection in Multiple-class Classification 130
  5.7.1 Estimation of the generalized Youden index and respective cut-off points 131
  5.7.2 Euclidean distance from the perfection corner to obtain optimized cut-offs in the 3-class setting 133
5.8 Further Topics in Three- and k-class ROC Methodology 135
5.9 Exercises 136

DOI: 10.1201/9780429170140-5

5.1 The ROC Surface for Ordered Three-class Classification

Notions of ROC curve analysis have been extended to accommodate problems of three-class and multiple-class classification, that is, to the general case of a categorical reference standard with more than two categories. The ROC surface has been proposed as a natural generalisation of the ROC curve for the assessment of diagnostic markers in three-class classification problems. The *Volume Under the ROC Surface (VUS)* is utilized as an index for the assessment of the diagnostic accuracy of the marker under consideration (see e.g. Nakas (2014) [185] for an overview of the topic).

ROC surface analysis is a valuable tool for three-class classification problems as it naturally generalizes ROC curve analysis within the ROC theoretical framework. The utility of ROC surface analysis is demonstrated by the numerous applications that have appeared in diverse subdisciplines in Medicine, such as Cardiology [100, 218], Neurology [42, 60, 267, 299], Opthalmology [54], Telecare [174], Nutrition [51, 74], Imaging [1], etc.; but also in areas of Bioinformatics, e.g. in -omics research [146,303] and Machine Learning [52,236,285].

A useful `R` package for the implementation of ROC surface analysis is `trinROC` [193] that can be downloaded from CRAN. Implementation of procedures supported by the `trinROC` package will also be discussed in this chapter. A user-friendly `python` package offering some of the features of `trinROC` also exists [154].

5.1.1 The three-class model

To fix ideas, we first consider the setting in which a reference standard exists categorizing subjects into one of three categories or classes, denoted as classes 1, 2, and 3. The data consist of n_1 marker values from class 1, denoted by X_1, which follow a continuous distribution with cdf F_1 (i.e. $X_1 \sim F_1$), and similarly for n_2 marker values from class 2, $X_2 \sim F_2$, and for n_3 marker values from class 3, $X_3 \sim F_3$. For simplicity of notation, we dropped the subscript for subject here. A decision rule that classifies subjects in one of these classes can be defined using two ordered threshold points $c_1 < c_2$ on the common continuous scale of the observations. For example, if the ordering of interest is $X_1 < X_2 < X_3$, the decision rule is illustrated graphically in Figure 5.1. The researcher's goal is the assessment of the ability of a diagnostic marker in correctly classifying subjects from the three ordered classes.

The construction of the corresponding ROC *surface* is based on the following algorithm:

- Step 1: Decide for class 1 when a measurement is less than c_1;
- Step 2: Decide for class 2 when it is between c_1 and c_2;
- Step 3: Decide for class 3 otherwise.

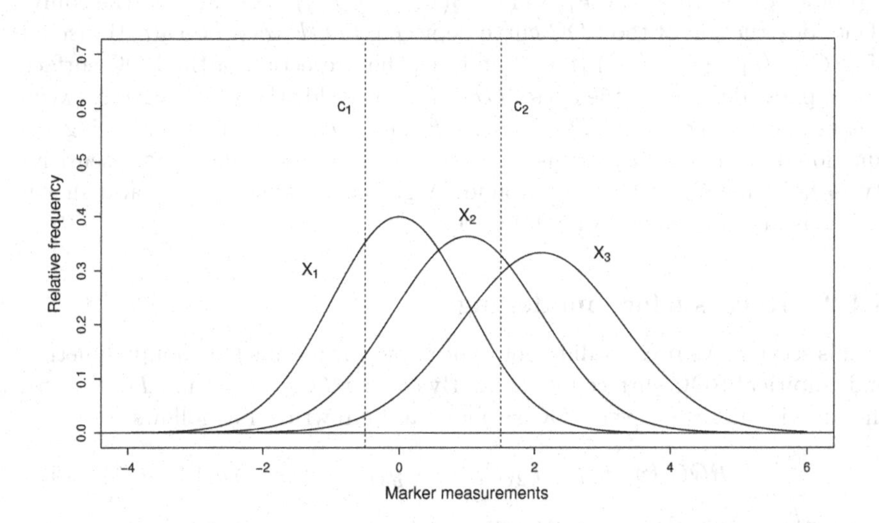

FIGURE 5.1
The three-class classification problem for $X_1 < X_2 < X_3$. The decision is driven by the choice of c_1 and c_2. The overlap in the underlying distributions results in three possible True- and six possible False- Class Fractions.

For a pair of cut-off points (c_1, c_2), this decision rule will result in three True Class Fractions (TCF) and six False Class Fractions (FCF) as follows: $TCF_1 = P(X_1 \leq c_1)$, $TCF_2 = P(c_1 < X_2 \leq c_2)$, and $TCF_3 = P(X_3 > c_2)$. Also, $FCF_{12} = P(c_1 \leq X_1 \leq c_2)$ and the remaining five possible FCF_{ij}, $i, j = 1, 2, 3$, $i \neq j$ are defined accordingly.

Notice that, TCF_1 is the probability that a measurement from class 1 will be classified correctly according to the ROC surface construction algorithm and similarly for TCF_2 and TCF_3, while FCF_{ij} is the probability that a measurement from class i will be erroneously classified as belonging to class j.

The ROC surface is defined as the set of triplets (TCF_1, TCF_2, TCF_3) which are obtained by varying c_1, c_2 in the union of the supports of F_1, F_2, and F_3, while keeping the order $c_1 < c_2$ fixed, The TCF take values in $[0, 1]$ with corner coordinates $\{(1, 0, 0),\ (0, 1, 0),\ (0, 0, 1)\}$. Thus, the ROC surface is the three-dimensional plot in the unit cube depicting $(F_1(c_1), F_2(c_2) - F_2(c_1), 1 - F_3(c_2))$, for all cut-off points (c_1, c_2), with $c_1 < c_2$. The functional form of the ROC surface is [190]:

$$ROC_s(TCF_1, TCF_3) = F_2(F_3^{-1}(1 - TCF_3)) - F_2(F_1^{-1}(TCF_1)).$$

It can be shown that this is a generalization of the ROC curve in three dimensions since projecting the ROC surface to the plane defined by TCF_2 versus TCF_1, i.e. setting $TCF_3 = 0$, the ROC curve between classes 1 and 2 is produced, i.e. $ROC(TCF_1) = 1 - F_2(F_1^{-1}(TCF_1))$. The latter is the equivalent construction of the ROC curve depicting $(TCF_1(c_1), TCF_2(c_1))$ instead of $(FCF_{12}(c_1), TCF_2(c_1))$ [190]. Similarly, the projection of the ROC surface to the plane defined by the axes TCF_2, TCF_3, yields the ROC curve between classes 2 and 3, i.e. $ROC(TCF_3) = F_2(F_3^{-1}(1 - TCF_3))$, the latter being the functional form of TCF_2 versus TCF_3 analogous to specificity versus sensitivity rather than the other way around. A graphical illustration is also shown in Nakas and Yiannoutsos (2004) [190].

5.1.2 ROC surface modelling

In this section, we present different approaches for parametric, nonparametric, and empirical ROC surface modeling. By setting $TCF_1 = p_1$ and $TCF_3 = p_3$, the functional form of the ROC surface can be rewritten as follows:

$$ROC_s(p_1, p_3) = F_2(F_3^{-1}(1 - p_3)) - F_2(F_1^{-1}(p_1)), \tag{5.1}$$

and $F_1^{-1}(p_1) \leq F_3^{-1}(1 - p_3)$. We will use this form of the ROC surface for the rest of the presentation.

5.1.2.1 Empirical and general nonparametric estimation

The empirical estimator of the ROC surface can be obtained by replacing the distribution functions in the definition of the ROC surface with their empirical counterparts. Thus, the empirical estimator of the ROC surface is

$$R\hat{O}C_s(p_1, p_3) = \hat{F}_2(\hat{F}_3^{-1}(1 - p_3)) - \hat{F}_2(\hat{F}_1^{-1}(p_1)),$$

where $\hat{F}_1, \hat{F}_2$, and $\hat{F}_3$ are the empirical distribution functions for the marker values from the three classes. In practice, we define

$$T\hat{C}F_1 = \frac{\Sigma_{i=1}^{n_1} I(X_{1i} < c_1)}{n_1},$$

$$T\hat{C}F_2 = \frac{\Sigma_{j=1}^{n_2} I(c_1 < X_{2j} < c_2)}{n_2},$$

$$T\hat{C}F_3 = \frac{\Sigma_{k=1}^{n_3} I(c_2 < X_{3k})}{n_3},$$

where $I(.)$ is the index function being equal to one if the expression in the brackets is true; otherwise, it is equal to zero. The derived $TCF_1(c_1, c_2)$, $TCF_2(c_1, c_2)$, $TCF_3(c_1, c_2)$ estimates provide the points defining the ROC surface for possible values of c_1, c_2 with $c_1 < c_2$.

In addition to empirical estimation, kernel-based and Bayesian methods have been proposed in the literature [131, 136]. In kernel-based approaches, estimates of F_1, F_2, and F_3, can be obtained via Gaussian kernel estimators of the form $\hat{F_i}(t) = \frac{1}{n_i}\Sigma_{j=1}^{n_i}\Phi(\frac{t - X_{ij}}{h_i})$, with $i = 1, 2, 3$. For the bandwidth h_i

which controls the amount of smoothing, Kang and Tian (2013) [136] have considered $h_i = (\frac{4}{3n_i})^{1/5} min(SD_i, IQR_i/1.349)$. SD_i and IQR_i are the standard deviation and interquartile range, respectively, for X_i measurements. This approach generalizes the two-class ROC curve framework in the three-class problem.

A Bayesian nonparametric method for the estimation of the ROC surface was proposed by Inácio et al. (2011) [131]. The method is based on Finite Polya Tree (FPT) hierarchical prior distributions for the three classes and involves the specification of independent FPT prior distributions for F_i, $i = 1, 2, 3$ conditional on a set of hyperparameters, i.e.:

$$F_i | c_i, \theta_i \sim FPT_{J_i}(F_{\theta_i}, c_i), \quad i = 1, 2, 3.$$

Suppose, F_i are centered at $F_{\boldsymbol{\theta}_i} = \mathrm{N}(\mu_i, \sigma_i)$, where $\boldsymbol{\theta}_i = (\mu_i, \sigma_i)$. The mixing parameters μ_i have independent normal prior distributions $\mathrm{N}(a_{\mu_i}, b_{\mu_i})$, whereas σ_i have independent gamma prior distributions $\Gamma(a_{\sigma_i}, b_{\sigma_i})$. Hyperparameters are considered fixed. The levels of the finite Polya trees determine the level of detail that is accommodated by the model and are set equal to J_i. Further details can be found in Inácio et al. (2011) [131].

5.1.2.2 Parametric estimation, the trinormal model

Parametric estimation of the ROC surface often makes use of the so-called trinormal model. Specifically, the trinormal model considers that marker values for each of the three classes follow a normal distribution or they can be transformed to normality through a common transformation. In the continuous marker case, an adapted version of the Box-Cox transformation is used for this purpose as will be described and illustrated later on in this section.

Under the normality assumptions for F_1, F_2, and F_3 (i.e. $X_1 \sim N(\mu_1, \sigma_1^2)$, $X_2 \sim N(\mu_2, \sigma_2^2)$, $X_3 \sim N(\mu_3, \sigma_3^2)$) the parametric form of the ROC surface is [294]:

$$ROC_s(p_1, p_3) = \Phi\left(\frac{\Phi^{-1}(1 - p_3) + d}{c}\right) - \Phi\left(\frac{\Phi^{-1}(p_1) + b}{a}\right),$$

with $\frac{\Phi^{-1}(p_1)+b}{a} \leq \frac{\Phi^{-1}(1-p_3)+d}{c}$. Φ is the distribution function of the standard normal distribution and $\boldsymbol{\beta} = (a, b, c, d)^t$ is a vector which specifies the parameters of the ROC surface. Under the normality assumption, components of $\boldsymbol{\beta}$ may be expressed as functions of the means and variances of F_1, F_2, and F_3, as follows:

$$a = \frac{\sigma_2}{\sigma_1}, \qquad b = \frac{\mu_1 - \mu_2}{\sigma_1}, \qquad c = \frac{\sigma_2}{\sigma_3}, \qquad d = \frac{\mu_3 - \mu_2}{\sigma_3}. \tag{5.2}$$

Estimation of an ROC surface using the trinormal model can be performed by estimating the parameters a, b, c and d using maximum likelihood estimators of the means, $\hat{\mu}_k = \sum_{i=1}^{n_k} X_{ki}/n_k$, and the variances $\hat{\sigma}_k^2 = \sum_{i=1}^{n_k} (X_{ki} - \hat{\mu}_i)^2/n_k$, for $k = 1, 2, 3$.

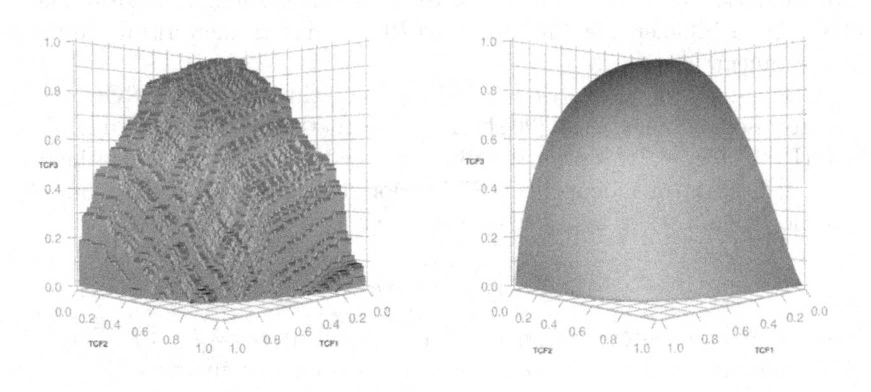

FIGURE 5.2
Empirical ROC surface (left panel) and corresponding parametric ROC surface based on the trinormal model (right panel).

Figure 5.2 illustrates an empirical ROC surface based on $n_1 = n_2 = n_3 =$ 100 marker values for each of three classes and the corresponding parametric estimate based on the trinormal model, directly assuming that the data are normally distributed. Data were simulated from underlying normal distributions and the `trinROC` package in `R` was used, as indicated below.

```
library(trinROC)
library(ggplot2)

markerx<-rnorm(100)
markery<-1+rnorm(100)
markerz<-1.8+rnorm(100)

rocsurf.emp(markerx,markery,markerz)   # left panel
rocsurf.trin(markerx,markery,markerz)     # right panel
```

Kang and Tian (2013) [136] applied a Box-Cox transformation for non-normally distributed data prior to fitting a parametric normal model. They then compared the results to those from a kernel-based estimate, in terms of bias and accuracy of the estimation of the Volume Under the ROC Surface (VUS) (see Section 5.1.2.1). The two-class Box-Cox transformation in the ROC curve framework was described in Section 3.1.1.1. Its generalization to the three-class case makes use of the following profile likelihood for the estimation of the transformation parameter λ:

$$l(\lambda) = -\frac{n_1}{2}\log[\frac{\Sigma_{j=1}^{n_1}(X_{1j}^{(\lambda)} - \frac{\Sigma_{j=1}^{n_1} X_{1j}^{(\lambda)}}{n_1})^2}{n_1}] - \frac{n_2}{2}\log[\frac{\Sigma_{i=1}^{n_2}(X_{2i}^{(\lambda)} - \frac{\Sigma_{i=1}^{n_2} X_{2i}^{(\lambda)}}{n_2})^2}{n_2}]$$
$$+ -\frac{n_3}{2}\log[\frac{\Sigma_{k=1}^{n_3}(X_{3k}^{(\lambda)} - \frac{\Sigma_{k=1}^{n_3} X_{3k}^{(\lambda)}}{n_3})^2}{n_3}]$$
$$+ (\lambda - 1)(\Sigma_{j=1}^{n_1}\log X_{1j} + \Sigma_{i=1}^{n_2}\log X_{2i} + \Sigma_{k=1}^{n_3}\log X_{3k}) + c$$

where c is constant and $X_1^{(\lambda)}$, $X_2^{(\lambda)}$, $X_3^{(\lambda)}$ are the transformed measurements. The procedure can be readily implemented using the `trinROC` package in R. We illustrate this here using marker A1GL measurements from the Pancreatic carcinoma data, described in Section 1.4.3.

```
library(trinROC)

#A1GL marker
a1glx<-ca199noll$A1GL[ca199noll$Group==2]
a1glx<-a1glx[-c(9,27)] #removing missing values
a1gly<-ca199noll$A1GL[ca199noll$Group==7]
a1glz<-ca199noll$A1GL[ca199noll$Group==1]
norma1gl<-boxcoxROC(a1glx,a1gly,a1glz)
```

```
## ---------------------------------------------------------------------
## Optimal lambda       = 0.3
## Shift param. lambda2 = 0

## Shapiro p-values for original data:
## x = 0.8018255, y = 0.02880135, z = 0.007114873

## Shapiro p-values for Box-Cox transformed data:
## x = 0.3958215, y = 0.4302764, z = 0.0764487
## ---------------------------------------------------------------------
```

Transformed measurements can be directly used for the construction of the parametric ROC surface under the trinormal model. The `boxcoxROC` function in `trinROC` provides the transformation parameter λ and an assessment for the normality assumption before and after the transformation, along with an object comprising the transformed measurements.

Under the Bayesian parametric paradigm, in order to find estimates of the beta parameters, an MCMC approach is needed. A Metropolis–Hastings algorithm or a Gibbs sampler can be employed. The use of the Metropolis–Hastings algorithm with uninformative normal priors for the means and uninformative gamma prior distributions for the standard deviations is described in Inácio et al. (2011) [131].

5.2 The Volume Under the ROC Surface (VUS) and its Estimation

The Volume Under the ROC Surface (VUS) is an analog of the AUC and is defined as

$$VUS = \int_0^1 \int_0^{1-F_3(F_1^{-1}(p_1))} ROC_s(p_1, p_3) dp_3 dp_1.$$

The theoretical VUS is equal to $P(X_1 < X_2 < X_3)$ [181]. An unbiased non-parametric estimator of VUS is given by

$$\hat{VUS} = \frac{1}{n_1 n_2 n_3} \sum_{i=1}^{n_1} \sum_{j=1}^{n_2} \sum_{k=1}^{n_3} I(X_{1i}, X_{2j}, X_{3k}),$$

where $I(X_1, X_2, X_3)$ equals one if X_1, X_2, X_3 are in the correct order and zero otherwise [73]. The definition of $I(X_1, X_2, X_3)$ can be adapted in order to adjust for the presence of ties. Specifically, when ties are present, define: $I(X_1, X_2, X_3) = \frac{1}{2}$ if $X_1 = X_2 < X_3$ or if $X_1 < X_2 = X_3$ and $I(X_1, X_2, X_3) = \frac{1}{6}$ if $X_1 = X_2 = X_3$, and $I(X_1, X_2, X_3) = 0$ (or 1 if perfectly ordered) otherwise. The expected value of VUS will then equal to

$$P(X_1 < X_2 < X_3) + \frac{1}{2} P(X_1 < X_2 = X_3) + \frac{1}{2} P(X_1 = X_2 < X_3) + \frac{1}{6} P(X_1 = X_2 = X_3).$$

VUS takes the value $\frac{1}{3!} = \frac{1}{6}$ when the three distributions completely overlap and the value one when the three classes are perfectly separated in the correct order.

A parametric estimate of VUS can be obtained as follows [293]:

$$\hat{VUS} = \int\int_{\mathcal{A}} \Phi\left(\frac{\Phi^{-1}(1-p_3) + \hat{d}}{\hat{c}}\right) - \Phi\left(\frac{\Phi^{-1}(p_1) + \hat{b}}{\hat{a}}\right) dp_1 dp_3,$$

where $\mathcal{A} = \{(p_1, p_3) \,|\, 0 \le p_1 \le 1, 0 \le p_3 \le \Phi((\hat{\mu}_3 - \hat{\mu}_1 \cdot \hat{\sigma}_1 \cdot \Phi^{-1}(p_1)))/\hat{\sigma}_3)\}$.

Kang and Tian (2013) [136] report an extensive study comparing possible parametric and nonparametric approaches for the estimation of VUS in terms of bias and RMSE and support the use of kernel-based estimation in the general case.

In several situations in practice, researchers may wish to limit the study of the ROC surface to a clinically relevant range of measurement values. In such cases, the *partial VUS* has been defined [293]. The partial VUS generalizes the notion of the partial AUC from the general ROC curve framework in the two-class case. Other measures for the evaluation of the discrimination ability of a marker rising from the definition of the ROC surface has also been proposed in the literature. The interested reader is referred to the articles by Van Calster et al. (2012) [271,272].

Illustration of the estimation of the VUS via the `trinROC` package will be described in the next two sections.

5.3 Hypothesis Testing for VUS

5.3.1 Hypothesis testing for a single VUS

Formal assessment of the diagnostic accuracy of a marker in a three-class classification problem via its VUS can be based on testing the null hypothesis $H_0 : VUS = \frac{1}{6}$ versus the alternative of interest. This is the analog of testing for the $H_0 : AUC = \frac{1}{2}$ in the two-class case, given that there are six possible orderings in the three-class case (while only two in the two-class case).

A nonparametric test statistic for H_0 is given by

$$Z_1 = \frac{\hat{VUS} - \frac{1}{6}}{\sqrt{Var(\hat{VUS})}} \sim N(0,1). \qquad (5.3)$$

$\hat{VUS}$ is the nonparametric estimate of VUS. Then, Z_1 is asymptotically normally distributed based on results from U-statistics theory [145, 204]. The variance of $\hat{VUS}$ can be estimated by using U-statistics methodology or the bootstrap [190]. The bootstrap approach consists of sampling with replacement, n_1, n_2, n_3 subjects from the initial samples from X_1, X_2, X_3, respectively, and calculating the VUS for each of the b replications of this procedure. The bootstrap estimate of the variance of VUS is the sample variance of the b bootstrap values of VUS [190].

Properties of nonparametric estimators of the variance of $\hat{VUS}$ have been studied by Guangming et al. (2013) [99]. Based on Z_1, 95% confidence intervals for VUS can be constructed in a straightforward fashion. Wan (2012) [282] proposed an empirical likelihood confidence interval for the nonparametric estimate of VUS.

A parametric approach for confidence interval construction for VUS was discussed by Xiong et al. (2006) [293]. Confidence intervals are constructed based on the delta method. Alternatively, the bootstrap can be used again, where for each bootstrap replication the parametric VUS is calculated. Non-parametric predictive inference for the ROC surface and the VUS is developed in Coolen-Maturi et al. (2013) [58].

The function `roc.eda` in `trinROC` with the option `"type = empirical"` provides an empirical estimate of the VUS and formally tests its significance using the bootstrap. Performance of the A1GL marker from the pancreatic cancer dataset is illustrated here.

```
library(trinROC)

roc.eda(a1glx,a1gly,a1glz, type="empirical")
```

```
## Data overview of empirical ROC Classifier
## ---------------------------------------------------------------------

## Applied test: Bootstrap test
## Significance level: 0.05
## Alternative hypothesis: two.sided
## ---------------------------------------------------------------------
## data: a1glx, a1gly and a1glz

## Boot statistic: 4.718, Boot p.value: 0

## empirical VUS:  0.475
## ---------------------------------------------------------------------
```

The results of this analysis show that A1GL is a statistically significant marker in discriminating between the three classes: “normal”, “pancreatitis”, “pancreatic cancer”, in the sense that, using A1GL to discriminate between the three classes in the anticipated order is better than chance allocation. More elaborate hypotheses can be tested as well, e.g. setting a lower pre-defined limit for the VUS value that would be clinically relevant. The only “twist” would be to replace $\frac{1}{6}$ in the nominator of Equation (5.3) with the predefined value. The Z_1 statistic is equal to 4.718. One may then calculate the denominator in Equation (5.3) to be equal to 0.065 in a straightforward manner. An approximate 95% confidence interval for the empirical VUS can be calculated by adding and subtracting in turn 2×0.065 to the VUS estimate. Thus, $\hat{\text{VUS}}$=0.475, (95% CI: $0.345, 0.605$).

5.3.2 Comparison of diagnostic markers via their VUS estimates

As in the case of the AUC, the Volume Under the ROC Surface can be used to compare diagnostic markers. To fix ideas, we consider an example in which two markers (A and B) are measured on the same $n = n_1 + n_2 + n_3$ specimens which are classified by a gold standard procedure into three ordered disease classes. Let (X_1^A, X_2^A, X_3^A) and (X_1^B, X_2^B, X_3^B) be the values for markers A and B, respectively.

In order to compare VUS^A and VUS^B via their nonparametric, empirical estimates, Dreiseitl et al. (2000) [73] proposed a U-statistics approach. Specifically, the null hypothesis $H_0 : VUS^A = VUS^B$ is tested by calculating

$$Z_2 = \frac{\hat{VUS}^A - \hat{VUS}^B}{\sqrt{Var(\hat{VUS}^A) + Var(\hat{VUS}^B) - 2 \cdot Cov(\hat{VUS}^A, \hat{VUS}^B)}}$$

and then comparing this value to a standard normal distribution. Alternatively, the bootstrap can be used to test H_0 [190].

The latter procedure can be directly implemented in R using the trinROC package for the comparison of markers A1GL and CA19-9 via their empirical VUS estimates as follows:

```
library(trinROC)

roc.eda(a1glx,a1gly,a1glz, scatter=T, type="empirical")
roc.eda(ca199markx, ca199marky, ca199markz, type="empirical")
# results from the two lines of code above not shown here

boot.test(a1glx,a1gly,a1glz,
ca199markx, ca199marky, ca199markz, paired = TRUE)
```

```
## Bootstrap test for comparison of two independent classifiers
##
## data:  a1glx a1gly a1glz and ca199markx ca199marky ca199markz
## Z-stat = -0.9391, p-value = 0.3477
## alternative hypothesis: true Difference in VUS is not equal to 0
## sample estimates:
## VUS of Classifier 1 VUS of Classifier 2
##           0.4749747           0.5654858
```

We conclude that the two markers do not differ significantly in separating non-diseased subjects, pancreatitis patients, and pancreatic cancer patients based on VUS estimates of their corresponding empirical ROC surfaces.

Xiong et al. (2007) [294] studied the parametric analogue for the comparison of VUSs based on the results in Xiong et al. (2006) [293], while Tian et al. (2011) [257] considered the parametric approach using notions of generalized pivots. We note that direct use of the trinormal model when normality assumptions does not hold usually underestimates the VUS.

The method of Xiong et al. (2007) [294] is implemented in the `trinROC` package. The comparison of markers A1GL and CA19-9 via their trinormal model-based VUS estimates is as follows:

```
trinVUS.test(a1glx,a1gly,a1glz,
ca199markx, ca199marky, ca199markz, paired = TRUE)
```

```
##  Trinormal VUS test for comparison of paired ROC data

## data:  a1glx a1gly a1glz and ca199markx ca199marky ca199markz
## Z-stat = -0.32541, p-value = 0.7449
## alternative hypothesis: true Difference in VUS is not equal to 0
## sample estimates:
## VUS of Classifier 1 VUS of Classifier 2
##           0.4450707           0.4719855
```

5.4 Hypothesis Testing for the Entire ROC Surface

5.4.1 Comparing two markers

ROC curves and surfaces can be compared in their entirety or on the basis of summary measures such as the area under the curve or the volume under the surface. Parametric and nonparametric methods for comparing entire curves were discussed in Section 4.3.4. In particular Metz and Kronman (1980) [171] proposed a test to compare two ROC curves from unpaired data. The test is based on a binormal model assumption and used only the parameters of the model. A similar test for paired data is also available [173]. This concept has been adapted in the three-class setting (under the ROC surface framework) and a test statistic based on the parameters of the trinormal model-based ROC surface given in Equation (5.2) has been proposed in Noll et al. (2019) [193].

To fix ideas, consider the comparison of two markers (denoted as Classifier k, for $k = 1, 2$ in the `trinROC` package; slightly changing the notation relative to other sections of marker comparisons in this book) using the corresponding ROC surfaces estimated via the trinormal model. The estimates

$(\hat{a}_k, \hat{b}_k, \hat{c}_k, \hat{d}_k)^T$ of the parameters in the trinormal model can be obtained from Equation (5.2). Dorfman and Alf show that, for the binormal ROC model, the parameter estimates follow a multivariate normal distribution. This result extends to the ROC surface under the trinormal assumption [193].

The null hypothesis for the comparison of ROC surfaces is $H_0: a_1 = a_2,\ b_1 = b_2,\ c_1 = c_2, d_1 = d_2$ and the alternative hypothesis is H_A: $a_1 \neq a_2$ or $b_1 \neq b_2$ or $c_1 \neq c_2$ or $d_1 \neq d_2$. The test statistic is approximately chi-squared distributed with four degrees of freedom and can be written as:

$$X^2 = \begin{pmatrix} \hat{a}_1 - \hat{a}_2 & \hat{b}_1 - \hat{b}_2 & \hat{c}_1 - \hat{c}_2 & \hat{d}_1 - \hat{d}_2 \end{pmatrix} \widehat{W}^{-1} \begin{pmatrix} \hat{a}_1 - \hat{a}_2 \\ \hat{b}_1 - \hat{b}_2 \\ \hat{c}_1 - \hat{c}_2 \\ \hat{d}_1 - \hat{d}_2 \end{pmatrix}, \tag{5.4}$$

where, for unpaired data, $\widehat{W} = \widehat{W}_1 + \widehat{W}_2$ is the sum of the covariance matrices of the trinormal model parameters estimates $\hat{a}_k$, $\hat{b}_k$, $\hat{c}_k$, and $\hat{d}_k$. Specifically, these covariance matrices have the form

$$\widehat{W}_k = \begin{pmatrix} \sigma^2_{a_k} & \sigma_{a_k b_k} & \sigma_{a_k c_k} & \sigma_{a_k d_k} \\ \sigma_{b_k a_k} & \sigma^2_{b_k} & \sigma_{b_k c_k} & \sigma_{b_k d_k} \\ \sigma_{c_k a_k} & \sigma_{c_k b_k} & \sigma^2_{c_k} & \sigma_{c_k d_k} \\ \sigma_{d_k a_k} & \sigma_{d_k b_k} & \sigma_{d_k c_k} & \sigma^2_{d_k} \end{pmatrix}, \quad k = 1, 2.$$

The entries are obtained via the delta method

$$\widehat{W}_k = \begin{pmatrix} \frac{\hat{a}_k^2}{2}\left(\frac{1}{n_2} + \frac{1}{n_1}\right) & \frac{\hat{a}_k \hat{b}_k}{2n_1} & \frac{\hat{a}_k \hat{c}_k}{2n_2} & 0 \\ \frac{\hat{a}_k \hat{b}_k}{2n_1} & \frac{\hat{b}_k^2}{2n_1} + \frac{\hat{a}_k^2}{n_2} + \frac{1}{n_1} & 0 & \frac{\hat{a}_k \hat{c}_k}{n_2} \\ \frac{\hat{a}_k \hat{c}_k}{2n_2} & 0 & \frac{\hat{c}_k^2}{2}\left(\frac{1}{n_2} + \frac{1}{n_3}\right) & \frac{\hat{c}_k \hat{d}_k}{2n_3} \\ 0 & \frac{\hat{a}_k \hat{c}_k}{n_2} & \frac{\hat{c}_k \hat{d}_k}{2n_3} & \frac{\hat{d}_k^2}{2n_3} + \frac{\hat{c}_k^2}{n_2} + \frac{1}{n_3} \end{pmatrix}, \ k=1,2. \tag{5.5}$$

The null hypothesis will be rejected if $X^2 > \chi^2_\alpha$, where χ^2_α is the appropriate quantile of the chi-squared distribution with four degrees of freedom.

When the marker measurements are unpaired, the estimated parameters $\hat{a}_1, \hat{b}_1, \hat{c}_1, \hat{d}_1$ are independent from $\hat{a}_2, \hat{b}_2, \hat{c}_2, \hat{d}_2$, and hence all the covariance terms for estimates between the two ROC surfaces are zero. As a consequence, $\widehat{W}$ can be written as the sum of the covariances of the two sets of parameters.

When the marker measurements are paired, the test statistic can be written as

$$X^2 = \begin{pmatrix} \hat{a}_1 - \hat{a}_2 & \hat{b}_1 - \hat{b}_2 & \hat{c}_1 - \hat{c}_2 & \hat{d}_1 - \hat{d}_2 \end{pmatrix} \widehat{W^*}^{-1} \begin{pmatrix} \hat{a}_1 - \hat{a}_2 \\ \hat{b}_1 - \hat{b}_2 \\ \hat{c}_1 - \hat{c}_2 \\ \hat{d}_1 - \hat{d}_2 \end{pmatrix} \tag{5.6}$$

and follows approximately a chi-squared distribution with four degrees of freedom. Using the delta method, the entries of the 4×4 symmetric $\widehat{W}^*$ matrix are derived as follows:

$$
\begin{aligned}
\widehat{w}^*_{11} &= \frac{a_1^2}{2}\left(\frac{1}{n_2}+\frac{1}{n_1}\right)+\frac{a_2^2}{2}\left(\frac{1}{n_2}+\frac{1}{n_1}\right)-2\left(\frac{\widehat{\rho}_2^2 a_1 a_2}{2n_2}+\frac{\widehat{\rho}_1^2 a_1 a_2}{2n_1}\right),\\
\widehat{w}^*_{12} &= \frac{a_1 b_1}{2n_1}+\frac{a_2 b_2}{2n_1}-\frac{a_1 b_2 \widehat{\rho}_1}{2n_1}-\frac{a_2 b_1 \widehat{\rho}_1}{2n_1},\\
\widehat{w}^*_{13} &= \frac{a_1 c_1}{2n_2}+\frac{a_2 c_2}{2n_2}-\frac{a_1 c_2 \widehat{\rho}_2}{2n_2}-\frac{a_2 c_1 \widehat{\rho}_2}{2n_2},\\
\widehat{w}^*_{22} &= \frac{b_1^2}{2n_1}+\frac{a_1^2}{n_2}+\frac{1}{n_1}+\frac{b_2^2}{2n_1}+\frac{a_2^2}{n_2}+\frac{1}{n_1}-2\left(\frac{\widehat{\rho}_1^2 b_1 b_2}{2n_2}+\frac{\widehat{\rho}_2^2 a_1 a_2}{n_2}+\frac{\widehat{\rho}_1}{n_1}\right),\\
\widehat{w}^*_{24} &= \frac{a_1 c_1}{n_2}+\frac{a_2 c_2}{n_2}-\frac{a_1 c_2 \widehat{\rho}_2}{n_2}-\frac{a_2 c_1}{n_2},\\
\widehat{w}^*_{33} &= \frac{c_1^2}{2}\left(\frac{1}{n_2}+\frac{1}{n_3}\right)+\frac{c_2^2}{2}\left(\frac{1}{n_2}+\frac{1}{n_3}\right)-2\left(\frac{\widehat{\rho}_2^2 c_1 c_2}{2n_2}+\frac{\widehat{\rho}_3^2 c_1 c_2}{2n_3}\right),\\
\widehat{w}^*_{34} &= \frac{c_1 d_1}{2n_3}+\frac{c_2 d_2}{2n_3}-\frac{c_1 d_2 \widehat{\rho}_3}{2n_3}-\frac{c_2 d_1 \widehat{\rho}_3}{2n_3},\\
\widehat{w}^*_{44} &= \frac{d_1^2}{2n_3}+\frac{c_1^2}{n_2}+\frac{1}{n_3}+\frac{d_2^2}{2n_3}+\frac{c_2^2}{n_2}+\frac{1}{n_3}-2\left(\frac{\widehat{\rho}_3^2 d_1 d_2}{2n_3}+\frac{\widehat{\rho}_2^2 c_1 c_2}{n_2}+\frac{\widehat{\rho}_3}{n_3}\right),\\
\widehat{w}^*_{14} &= \widehat{w}^*_{23} = 0,
\end{aligned}
$$

where $\widehat{\rho}_l$, $l = 1, 2, 3$, are the corresponding pairwise Pearson correlation coefficients of the marker measurements between the two markers for each group. We reject H_0, if $X^2 > \chi^2_\alpha$ just as we did in the unpaired case.

Implementation of the testing procedure can be done via the `trinROC` package in R. The following illustration uses synthetic data for two unpaired markers.

```
library(trinROC)

x1<-rnorm(50)
x2<-1+rnorm(50)
x3<-1.5+1.4*rnorm(50)
y1<-3+rnorm(50)
y2<-3.5+0.8*rnorm(50)
y3<-5+1.2*rnorm(50)

trinROC.test(x1,x2,x3, y1,y2,y3, paired = FALSE)
# use paired = TRUE when both markers
# are measured on the same individuals
```

```
## Trinormal based ROC test for comparison of two independent classifiers
```

```
## data:  x1 x2 x3 and y1 y2 y3
## Chi-Squared test = 17.575, df = 4, p-value = 0.001494
## alternative hypothesis: true a1-a2, b1-b1, c1-c2 and d1-d2 is not equal to 0
## sample estimates:
##                     VUS        a          b         c         d
## Classifier1: 0.3594287 1.115649 -0.9011437 0.9083820 0.2847709
## Classifier2: 0.5499377 1.054275 -0.6605672 0.8045092 1.3926547
```

The software also accommodates the analysis of data from paired markers. Implementation is left as an exercise in Section 5.9.

5.4.2 Box-Cox transformation when comparing two markers

If the trinormal model is not justified by the data at hand, we can use the Box-Cox transformation in a similar fashion to the two-class case. To proceed, one would need a Box-Cox transformation that will transform all measurements (from all three groups) generated by marker A, and a separate transformation that will transform the measurements of of marker B. The underlying transformation parameters are denoted with λ_A and λ_B, respectively. The corresponding likelihood was derived in Bantis and Feng (2018) [26] generalizing the two-class case in Molodianovitch et al. (2006) [176] and has the following form:

$$
\begin{aligned}
L(\mathbf{p}) = & \prod_{i=1}^{n_1} \frac{exp\left(-\frac{1}{2}\left(X_{1i}^A-\mu_{1(\lambda_A)}^A,\ X_{1i}^B-\mu_{1(\lambda_B)}^B\right)\boldsymbol{\Sigma}_1^{-1}\left(X_{1i}^A-\mu_{1(\lambda_A)}^A,\ X_{1i}^B-\mu_{1(\lambda_B)}^B\right)'\right)}{2\pi\sqrt{det(\boldsymbol{\Sigma}_1)}}\\
& \times \prod_{i=1}^{n_1} \frac{exp\left(-\frac{1}{2}\left(X_{2i}^A-\mu_2^A,\ X_{2i}^B-\mu_{2(\lambda_B)}^B\right)\boldsymbol{\Sigma}_2^{-1}\left(X_{2i}^A-\mu_{2(\lambda_A)}^A,\ X_{2i(\lambda_B)}^B-\mu_{2(\lambda_B)}^B\right)'\right)}{2\pi\sqrt{det(\boldsymbol{\Sigma}_2)}}\\
& \times \prod_{i=1}^{n_3} \frac{exp\left(-\frac{1}{2}\left(X_{3i}^A-\mu_{3(\lambda_A)}^A,\ X_{3i}^B-\mu_{3(\lambda_B)}^B\right)\boldsymbol{\Sigma}_3^{-1}\left(X_{3i}^A-\mu_{3(\lambda_A)}^A,\ X_{3i}^B-\mu_{3(\lambda_B)}^B\right)'\right)}{2\pi\sqrt{det(\boldsymbol{\Sigma}_3)}}\\
& \times \prod_{i=1}^{n_1}(X_{1i}^A)^{\lambda_A-1}\times\prod_{i=1}^{n_1}(X_{1i}^B)^{\lambda_B-1}\times\prod_{j=1}^{n_2}(X_{2j}^A)^{\lambda_A-1}\times\prod_{j=1}^{n_2}(X_{2j}^B)^{\lambda_B-1}\\
& \times \prod_{k=1}^{n_3}(X_{3k}^A)^{\lambda_A-1}\times\prod_{k=1}^{n_3}(X_{3k}^B)^{\lambda_B-1},
\end{aligned}
\tag{5.7}
$$

where

$$
\Sigma_1 = \begin{pmatrix} \left(\sigma_{1(\lambda_A)}^A\right)^2 & cov_1 \\ cov_1 & \left(\sigma_{1(\lambda_B)}^B\right)^2 \end{pmatrix}, \quad \Sigma_2 = \begin{pmatrix} \left(\sigma_{2(\lambda_A)}^A\right)^2 & cov_2 \\ cov_2 & \left(\sigma_{2(\lambda_B)}^B\right)^2 \end{pmatrix}
$$

and likewise for Σ_3. Here, the parameter vector $\mathbf{p}$ is

$$
\mathbf{p} = (\mu_{1(\lambda_A)}^A, \sigma_{1(\lambda_A)}^A, \ldots, \mu_{3(\lambda_A)}^A, \sigma_{3(\lambda_A)}^A, \mu_{3(\lambda_B)}^B, \sigma_{3(\lambda_B)}^B, cov_1, cov_2, cov_3, \lambda_A, \lambda_B).
$$

where $\theta^{(\lambda_{A,B})} = (\mu_{1A}^{(\lambda_A)}, \sigma_{1A}^{(\lambda_A)}, \ldots, \sigma_{3B}^{(\lambda_B)}, cov_1^{(\lambda_{A,B})}, cov_2^{(\lambda_{A,B})}, cov_3^{(\lambda_{A,B})})$.

Note that the likelihood now depends on 17 parameters, the original 15 plus two extra transformation parameters, λ_A and λ_B. After computing the transformed scores, one may proceed as in the standard trinormal setting [176].

We note that the variability of both transformation parameters is ignored in this approach and both λ_A and λ_B are considered as fixed at their estimated values. However, as shown in Bantis and Feng (2018) [26], taking into account the variability of the estimated parameters is crucial in order to attain appropriate size of the proposed test. This can be done via the delta method and using the appropriate covariance submatrices extracted from the full 15×15 covariance matrix. The derivation of the statistic Z^* in this context is straightforward, by recognizing that all partial derivatives involved can be found in closed form. Analytical expressions of all covariance matrices and partial derivatives are given in Bantis and Feng (2016) [25].

5.4.3 Special case: Assessment of a single marker

A simplification of the method for comparing ROC surfaces of two markers provides an approach to testing hypotheses about a single marker. A hypothesis of interest in this setting is whether the ROC surface of a marker differs from the chance plane, that is whether the marker performs better than allocation by chance. The null hypothesis can be written as

$$H_0 : a_1 = 1,\ b_1 = 0\ , c_1 = 1, d_1 = 0$$

and the corresponding test statistic is

$$\chi^2 = \begin{pmatrix} \hat{a}_1 - 1 & \hat{b}_1 & \hat{c}_1 - 1 & \hat{d}_1 \end{pmatrix} \widehat{W}_1^{-1} \begin{pmatrix} \hat{a}_1 - 1 \\ \hat{b}_1 \\ \hat{c}_1 - 1 \\ \hat{d}_1 \end{pmatrix}, \tag{5.8}$$

with $\widehat{W_1}$ defined as in Equation (5.5). It is straightforward to show that, under the null hypothesis, χ^2 follows approximately a chi-squared distribution with four degrees of freedom.

The Box-Cox normalized data for marker A1GL from Section 5.3.2 are used for the illustration that follows.

```
library(trinROC)

roc.eda(norma1gl$xbc,norma1gl$ybc,norma1gl$zbc, type="trinormal")
```

```
## Data overview of trinormal ROC Classifier
```

```
## ----------------------------------------------------------------------

## Applied tests: Trinormal based ROC and VUS test
## Significance level: 0.05
## Alternative hypothesis: two.sided
## ----------------------------------------------------------------------
## data: normalgl$xbc, normalgl$ybc and normalgl$zbc

## ROC test statistic: 50.448, ROC p.value: 0
## VUS test statistic:  5.022 ,  VUS p.value:  0

## trinormal VUS:  0.444

## Parameters:
##  a b c d
##  1.7671 -1.3709 0.8788 0.5946
## ----------------------------------------------------------------------
```

We conclude that marker A1GL significantly separates the distributions of measurements from the three classes under study, since the corresponding ROC surface is significantly different from the chance plane that corresponds to a non-informative marker where all three marker measurement distributions completely overlap.

5.5 The ROC Umbrella, Different Order Restrictions

The notion of the ROC surface has been generalized to accommodate cases with umbrella or tree orderings (i.e. $X_1 < X_3 > X_2$ or $X_2 > X_1 < X_3$ respectively) between the three classes under study in Nakas and Alonzo (2007) [186]. The ROC surface and VUS reviewed in the previous sections are not directly applicable when such orderings are of interest. Specifically, these approaches do not allow one to assess the ability of a marker to differentiate two disease classes from a third disease class without requiring a specific monotone order for the three disease classes under study. The derivation of an ROC umbrella surface for the tree ordering $X_2 > X_1 < X_3$ is described here; however, the derivation is analogous for the umbrella ordering.

From basic set theory, in the strictly continuous case, we have, $(X_2 > X_1 < X_3) = (X_1 < X_2 < X_3) \cup (X_1 < X_3 < X_2)$ or equivalently in probabilistic terms, $P(X_2 > X_1 < X_3) = P(X_1 < X_2 < X_3) + P(X_1 < X_3 < X_2)$. The construction of two ROC surfaces (say surface A, surface B) corresponding to the orderings $X_1 < X_2 < X_3$ and $X_1 < X_3 < X_2$, respectively, is possible. These are the plots of the points: $(TCF_1^A(c_1, c_2), TCF_2^A(c_1, c_2), TCF_3^A(c_1, c_2))$ and

$(TCF_1^B(c_1,c_2), TCF_2^B(c_1,c_2), TCF_3^B(c_1,c_2))$, respectively, with $(c_1,c_2) \in \mathbb{R}^2$ and $c_1 < c_2$.

The tree ordering can be viewed on a single graph in the unit cube by plotting on the same axes defined by $x = TCF_1^A$, $y = TCF_2^A$, $z = TCF_3^A$ in turn:

$$(TCF_1^A(c_1,c_2), TCF_2^A(c_1,c_2), TCF_3^A(c_1,c_2))$$

and

$$(1 - TCF_1^B(c_1,c_2), 1 - TCF_2^B(c_1,c_2), 1 - TCF_3^B(c_1,c_2))$$

with $(c_1,c_2) \in \mathbb{R}^2$ and $c_1 < c_2$. It can be shown by simple algebra that surfaces A, B, thus constructed on a single graph, are disjoint.

The resulting umbrella ROC graph is a diagnostic plot for the visual assessment of the degree of separation in the given ordering of the three populations based on the samples.

The volume under surface A plus the volume over surface B can be used for inference. We refer to this summary measure as the umbrella volume (UV). UV is equivalently the sum of the volumes under the ROC surfaces A and B corresponding to the monotone orderings $X_1 < X_2 < X_3$ and $X_1 < X_3 < X_2$, respectively. The umbrella ROC graph contains both ordered ROC surfaces.

The empirical, nonparametric, unbiased estimator of the volume of the umbrella ROC graph $P(X_2 > X_1 < X_3)$ is

$$\widehat{UV} = \frac{1}{n_1 n_2 n_3} \sum_{i=1}^{n_1} \sum_{j=1}^{n_2} \sum_{k=1}^{n_3} I_U(X_{1i}, X_{2j}, X_{3k}),$$

where $I_U(X_1, X_2, X_3)$ equals one if $X_2 > X_1 < X_3$ and zero otherwise. UV varies from zero to one and is equal to $P(X_1 < X_2 < X_3)+P(X_1 < X_3 < X_2) = \frac{1}{6}+\frac{1}{6}=\frac{1}{3}$, when the three distributions completely overlap and equals one when the three classes are perfectly discriminated in the given ordering. Figure 5.3 depicts the ROC umbrella graph in the case of an informative and an uninformative marker.

The variance of the UV can be obtained using:

$$Var(\hat{UV}) = Var(V\hat{U}S_A) + Var(V\hat{U}S_B) - 2 \cdot Cov(V\hat{U}S_A, V\hat{U}S_B) \quad (5.9)$$

In practice, for the observed data, ties may occur between measurements in the three disease classes, in which case $I_U(X_1, X_2, X_3)=1$ if $X_1 < X_2 = X_3$, $I_U(X_1, X_2, X_3)=\frac{1}{2}$ if $X_1 = X_2 < X_3$ or if $X_1 = X_3 < X_2$, and $I_U(X_1, X_2, X_3)=\frac{1}{6}$ if $X_1 = X_2 = X_3$. The expected value of UV will then be

$$\begin{aligned} &P(X_1 < X_2 < X_3) + P(X_1 < X_3 < X_2) + P(X_1 < X_2 = X_3) \\ &+\frac{1}{2}P(X_1 = X_2 < X_3) + \frac{1}{2}P(X_1 = X_3 < X_2) + \frac{1}{6}P(X_1 = X_2 = X_3). \end{aligned}$$

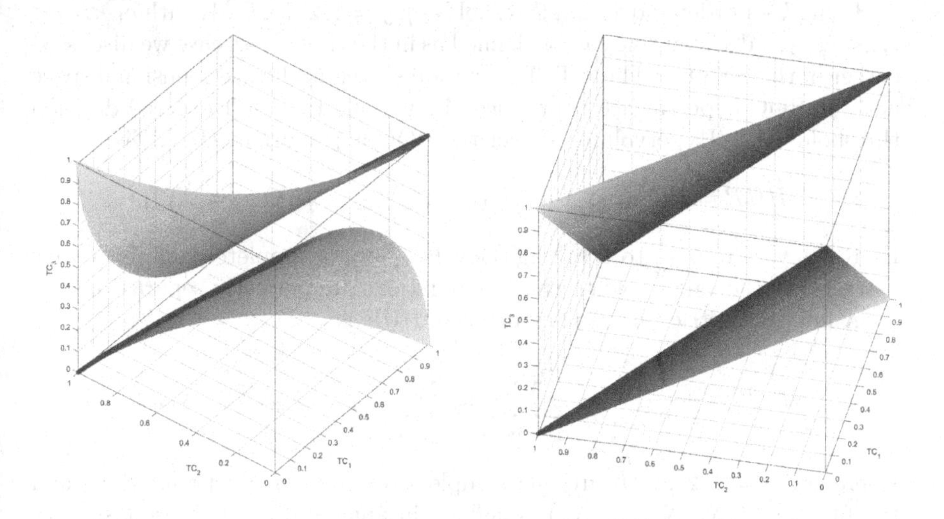

FIGURE 5.3
Left: The umbrella ROC graph for the configuration $X_1 \sim N(1, 1^2)$, $X_2 \sim N(3, 1^2)$, $X_3 \sim N(3.05, 1^2)$ after considering $X_2 > X_1 < X_3$. Right: An example of the umbrella ROC graph when the marker is uninformative and all three groups follow the same distribution. The volume under surface A and the volume above surface B' are both equal to $1/6$, thus yielding an umbrella volume (UV) equal to $1/3$.

Comparison of umbrella ROC volumes in a nonparametric framework has been studied in Alonzo and Nakas (2007) [4]. Alonzo et al. (2009) [5] provide a comparison of tests for restricted orderings in the three-class case, illustrating the usefulness of ROC surfaces and ROC umbrellas in different applied contexts. A two-dimensional representation of the ROC umbrella was proposed by Wang et al. (2016) [286].

5.6 ROC Hypersurfaces, Multiple-class Classification

For the k-class problem, with $k > 3$ and a single diagnostic marker, an ROC hypersurface may be constructed as described in Nakas and Yiannoutsos (2004) [190]. The hypersurface is a generalization of the concept of an ordinary surface in three-dimensional space to the case of an n-dimensional space [27].

Using $k-1$ ordered decision thresholds c_j, $j = 1, 2 \ldots, k-1$, with $c_1 < c_2 < \ldots < c_{k-1}$, a decision rule can be defined as in the three-class case we discussed earlier in this chapter. The k TCFs are represented in the k-dimensional space and the ROC hypersurface is produced by varying the $k-1$ ordered decision thresholds. The Hypervolume Under the ROC hypersurface (HUR) is

$$HUR = P((X_1 < X_2) \cap (X_2 < X_3) \cap \ldots \cap (X_{k-1} < X_k))$$

HUR will vary from $\frac{1}{k!}$ to 1, taking the value $\frac{1}{k!}$ for a completely uninformative marker and the value 1 when the k populations are perfectly separated.

A nonparametric unbiased estimate of HUR is

$$H\hat{U}R = \frac{1}{n_1 n_2 \ldots n_k} \sum_{i_1=1}^{n_1} \sum_{i_2=1}^{n_2} \ldots \sum_{i_k=1}^{n_k} I(X_{1i_1}, X_{2i_2}, \ldots, X_{ki_k}),$$

where n_i, $i = 1, 2, \ldots, k$ are the sample sizes from the k populations and the function $I(X_1, X_2, \ldots, X_k)$ is defined in analogy to the three-class case. Theoretical extensions relating to the general k-class problem are studied in Davidov and Herman (2012) [61].

5.7 Generalized Youden Index, Cut-off Point Selection in Multiple-class Classification

Similarly to the ROC curve, multiple-class generalizations of the Youden index have been proposed in the literature. A three-class Youden index for the assessment of accuracy and cut-off point selection in the three-class setting is discussed by Nakas et al. (2010) [187] and Nakas et al. (2013) [188]. Specifically, the proposed index has the following form:

$$\begin{aligned} J_3 &= max_{c_1, c_2; c_1 < c_2}\{TCF_1 + TCF_2 + TCF_3 - 1\} \\ &= max_{c_1, c_2; c_1 < c_2}\{F_1(c_1) + F_2(c_2) - F_2(c_1) - F_3(c_2)\}. \end{aligned} \tag{5.10}$$

The computation of J_3 involves constrained optimization with $c_1 < c_2$. This inequality will be true as long as the usual stochastic ordering of the form $P(X_1 > x) \leq P(X_2 > x) \leq P(X_3 > x)$ holds. In this case, J_3 is the sum of the Youden index for the two-class analysis of classes 1 and 2 and the Youden index for the two-class analysis of classes 2 and 3. The pair of cut-off points c_1, c_2 that corresponds to J_3 can be considered to be optimal in the sense of maximum accuracy and may be used in practice for decision-making in the three-class case. It follows that J_3 takes on values in $[0, 2]$. In order to restrict J_3 in $[0, 1]$, Luo and Xiong (2013) [159] have proposed the use of $\frac{J_3}{2}$.

Generalizing in k-class classification, given that the ordering of interest is $X_1 < \ldots < X_k$, the k-class Youden index is defined as follows:

$$J_{k;(1,2,\ldots,k-1)} = \sum_{i=1}^{k-1} J_{2;(i,i+1)} = J_{k-1;(1,2,\ldots,k-2)} + J_{2;(k-1,k)}. \tag{5.11}$$

That is, J_k is the sum of the Youden indices for the adjacent classes, when $c_1 < \ldots < c_{k-1}$. It is also the maximum vertical distance from the k-dimensional ROC hypersurface to the hyperplane defined by $TCF_1 + \ldots + TCF_k = 1$. J_k varies from zero when $F_1 = \ldots = F_k$, since all pairwise Youden indices are zero in that case, to $k-1$ when the class distributions are perfectly discriminated in the correct order, since all pairwise Youden indices will then be equal to one.

The generalized Youden index can serve as an index of the discriminatory ability of a diagnostic marker and further for the purpose of selecting the cut-off points that can be used for decision-making in practice. As in the two-class setting, weights can be added to the definition of J_3 to reflect the relative importance of the three TCFs. Use of a general cost function for the selection of cut-off points in multiple-class diagnostic testing has been studied in Skaltsa et al. [246]. Estimation and use of the generalized Youden index for nonparametric predictive inference is studied in Coolen-Maturi et al. (2013) [58]. An approach cut-off selection that accounts for misclassifications costs and for the prevalence of each group under a trichotomous setting is discussed in Bantis and Tsimikas (2022) [19].

5.7.1 Estimation of the generalized Youden index and respective cut-off points

J_3 can be estimated nonparametrically by using empirical distribution functions to obtain:

$$\begin{aligned} \hat{J}_3 &= max_{c_1,c_2;c_1<c_2}\{\hat{F}_1(c_1) + \hat{F}_2(c_2) - \hat{F}_2(c_1) - \hat{F}_3(c_2)\} \\ &= max_{c_1,c_2;c_1<c_2}\{\frac{\sum_{i=1}^{n_1} I(X_{1i} \leq c_1)}{n_1} - \frac{\sum_{j=1}^{n_2} I(X_{2j} \leq c_1)}{n_2} \\ &+ \frac{\sum_{j=1}^{n_2} I(X_{2j} \leq c_2)}{n_2} - \frac{\sum_{k=1}^{n_3} I(X_{3k} \leq c_2)}{n_3}\} \end{aligned} \tag{5.12}$$

where c_1 and c_2 are the empirical optimal cut-off values that result to the maximum value for the observed data. Numerically, the cut-off points are obtained by computing all possible values for J_3 and finding the maximum.

An alternative estimate can be obtained using kernel density estimation. In particular, a Gaussian kernel with bandwidth h_i, $i = 1, 2, 3$, respectively, gives rise to the following kernel-smoothed estimate of J_3:

$$\hat{J}_{3;KS} = max_{c_1,c_2;c_1<c_2}\{\frac{1}{n_1}\sum_{i=1}^{n_1}\Phi(\frac{c_1 - X_{1i}}{h_1}) - \sum_{j=1}^{n_2}\Phi(\frac{c_1 - X_{2j}}{h_2}) + \sum_{j=1}^{n_2}\Phi(\frac{c_2 - X_{2j}}{h_2}) - \sum_{k=1}^{n_3}\Phi(\frac{c_2 - X_{3k}}{h_3})\}. \quad (5.13)$$

As in the case of the nonparametric estimate of J_3, the optimal cut-off points c_1 and c_2 for the kernel density estimate are obtained by computing all possible values for J_3 and finding the maximum.

Parametric estimation of J_3 uses the particular distributional assumptions. In particular, under the assumption of normality, directly or after a Box-Cox transformation (see Section 5.1.2.2), the estimate is

$$J_3 = max_{c_1,c_2;c_1<c_2}\{\Phi(\frac{c_1 - \mu_1}{\sigma_1}) - \Phi(\frac{c_1 - \mu_2}{\sigma_2}) + \Phi(\frac{c_2 - \mu_2}{\sigma_2}) - \Phi(\frac{c_2 - \mu_3}{\sigma_3})\}. \quad (5.14)$$

The optimal cut-off points maximizing J_3 are obtained from :

$$c_1 = \frac{(\mu_2\sigma_1^2 - \mu_1\sigma_2^2) - \sigma_1\sigma_2\sqrt{(\mu_1 - \mu_2)^2 + (\sigma_1^2 - \sigma_2^2)log(\frac{\sigma_1^2}{\sigma_2^2})}}{\sigma_1^2 - \sigma_2^2} \quad (5.15)$$

$$c_2 = \frac{(\mu_3\sigma_2^2 - \mu_2\sigma_3^2) - \sigma_2\sigma_3\sqrt{(\mu_2 - \mu_3)^2 + (\sigma_2^2 - \sigma_3^2)log(\frac{\sigma_2^2}{\sigma_3^2})}}{\sigma_2^2 - \sigma_3^2}$$

The estimated values of the cut-off points require the estimates of the means and variances of the three markers. The reader should note that if $\sigma_1 = \sigma_2 = \sigma_3$, maximizing Equation (5.14) simplifies to $c_1 = \frac{\mu_1+\mu_2}{2}$ and $c_2 = \frac{\mu_2+\mu_3}{2}$.

Confidence intervals for J_3 can be constructed based on standard parametric or nonparametric bootstrap. Inference on differences of generalized Youden indices for the comparison of ROC surfaces has been studied in Yin et al. (2018) [300]. As in the three-class case, J_k can also be estimated nonparametrically by using the corresponding empirical distribution functions or parametrically based on distributional assumptions for the data.

Implementation of the parametric approach for cut-off point selection in the three-class case is supported by the `ThresholdROC` package in `R`. We will illustrate using marker A1GL after the Box-Cox transformation. One must keep in mind that estimated cut-offs refer to the transformed scale. Estimated values must be transformed back to the original scale in order to be used in practice. Figure 5.4 depicts smoothed estimates of the distributions of the three groups along with the corresponding cut-off points and respective confidence intervals. These results are also given in the corresponding output of the function `thres3`.

```
library(ThresholdROC)

rho <- c(1/3, 1/3, 1/3)
start <- c(mean(normalgl$xbc), mean(normalgl$zbc))
thr3 <- thres3(normalgl$xbc, normalgl$ybc, normalgl$zbc, rho,
   + dist1 = "norm", dist2 = "norm", dist3 = "norm",
   + start=start, ci.method = "boot")

plot(thr3, col = 1:4, lwd = c(2, 2, 2, 1), leg.po3s = "topright")

thr3
```

```
## Estimate:
##  Threshold 1:  0.6603414
##  Threshold 2:  0.9252874

## Confidence intervals (bootstrap):
##  CI based on normal distribution for Threshold 1:  0.5782241  -  0.7424587
##  CI based on percentiles for Threshold 1:  0.5659232  - 0.7317155
##  CI based on normal distribution for Threshold 2:  0.7125658  -  1.138009
##  CI based on percentiles for Threshold 2:  0.7011383  -  1.136884
##  Bootstrap resamples:  1000

# Parameters used:
##  Prevalences: 0.3333333 0.3333333 0.3333333
##  Costs
##    C11,C12,C13: 0 1 1
##    C21,C22,C23: 1 0 1
##    C31,C32,C33: 1 1 0
##  Significance Level:  0.05
```

5.7.2 Euclidean distance from the perfection corner to obtain optimized cut-offs in the 3-class setting

An alternative approach to derive optimal cut-off points is based on the Euclidean distance of the ROC surface to the perfection corner. The method has been described for trichotomous settings in Mosier and Bantis (2021) [178].

The Euclidean distance of the ROC surface from the perfection corner is defined as:

$$D^* = min_{c_1,c_2;c_1<c_2}\{(1-TCF_1)^2 + (1-TCF_2)^2 + (1-TCF_3)^2\}^{1/2}.$$

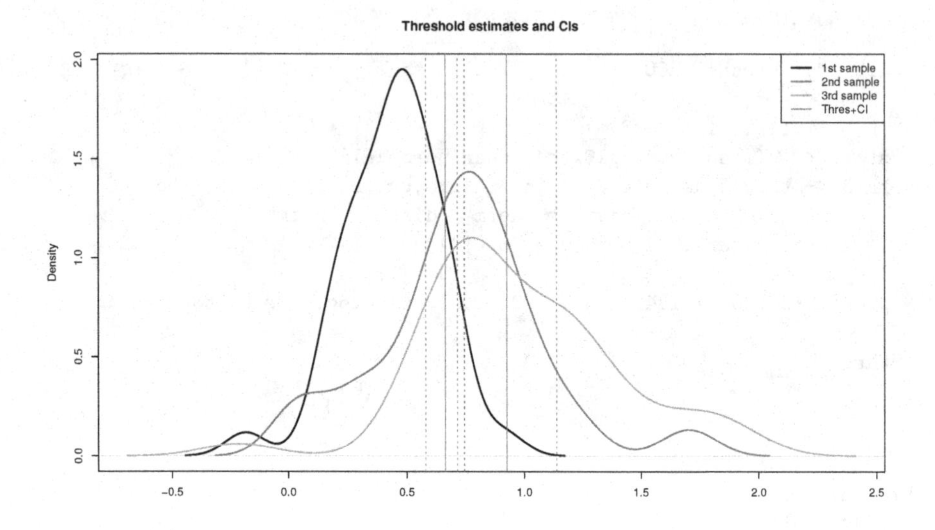

FIGURE 5.4
Cut-off point estimates along with corresponding confidence intervals using the `ThresholdROC` package.

The Euclidean distance from the perfection corner can be extended to the general k-class setting as follows:

$$D^* = min_{c_j;c_j<c_{j+1}}\left\{\sum_{i=1}^{k}(1-TCF_i)^2\right\}^{1/2}, j=1,...,k-1. \tag{5.16}$$

By minimizing this expression, we obtain estimates of the corresponding $k-1$ optimal cut-off values. A geometric representation of the differences between the generalized Youden index and the Euclidean distance from the perfection corner in the three-class setting is given in Figure 5.5.

Parametric and nonparametric methods for the relevant cut-off estimation are discussed in detail in Mosier and Bantis (2021) [178]. Their simulations show that, compared to the generalized Youden index, the Euclidean distance-based cut-offs exhibit tighter confidence intervals. The reason is that the Euclidean-based cut-offs are derived through the contribution of the biomarker scores from all three groups simultaneously. This is not the case for the three-class generalized Youden index for which, it turns out to be, cut-offs are actually obtained in a pairwise fashion. Euclidean-based cut-offs also involve smaller widths for the confidence intervals of the corresponding TCF triplets, compared to the Youden index-based ones [241]. Relevant `MATLAB` code for all methods can be found at `www.leobantis.net`.

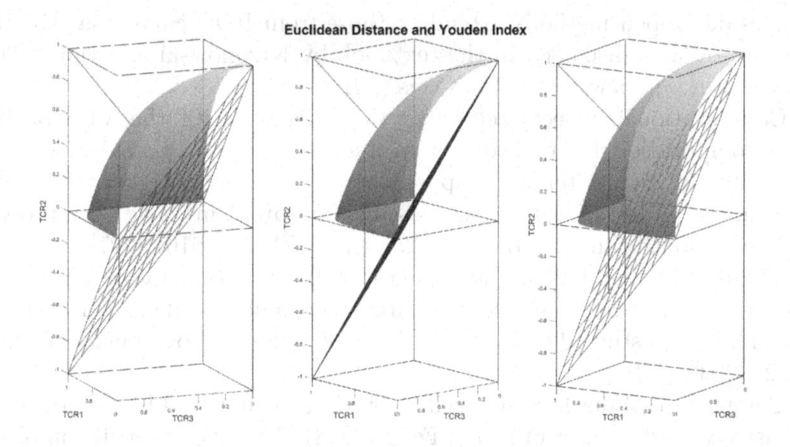

FIGURE 5.5
Plots comparing the Euclidean distance and the (generalized) Youden index of a biomarker score viewed from different perspectives for convenience. The Euclidean distance is represented by the red line segment while the generalized Youden index is represented by the blue line segment. The uninformative biomarker plane is represented by the diagonal gridded plane.

5.8 Further Topics in Three- and k-class ROC Methodology

The concept of the ROC surface was initially introduced by Scurfield (1996) [239]. However, the original paper received little attention in the literature, probably because it only described the theoretical construction of the ROC surface and did not discuss implementations and applications. A similar construction was proposed independently, a few years later, by Mossman (1999) [181] and was implemented in `Mathematica` by Heckerling (2001) [118].

Inference regarding the VUS using nonparametric statistics based on Mossman's construction was studied by Dreiseitl et al. (2000) [73]. The VUS is connected to nonparametric analogues of one-way ANOVA in the same way as the empirical AUC is connected to the Wilcoxon–Mann–Whitney statistic [5]. ROC surface construction and the generalization of this construction to multiple-class classification problems in a nonparametric context was consistently described in Nakas and Yiannoutsos (2004) [190]. The Nakas and Yannoutsos construction has been reintroduced by other authors later on (e.g. [149, 293]). In particular, Xiong et al. (2006) [293] explores extensively the parametric model, thus supplementing the work in Nakas and Yiannoutos (2004) [190]. Building on the fundamentals of the ROC surface, several authors developed methods extending those from ROC curve analysis. ROC surfaces are also discussed in the textbook by Krzanowski and Hand (2009) [143] and in a review article by Nakas (2014) [185].

Computational aspects regarding the calculation of the VUS or HUR when computational complexity is an issue have also appeared in the literature [52, 279, 280]. Alternative approaches for the generalization of the ROC curve in three- and multiple-class classification problems have been proposed by Yang and Carlin (2000) [296], Yang and Zhao (2010) [297], Hand and Till (2001) [103], and Wan and Zhang (2009) [283]. Generalizations of ROC analysis notions when the gold standard is continuous-scale rather than categorical has been studied by Obuchowski (2006) [199] and by Shiu and Gatsonis (2012) [243].

Comparison of markers at specific points of the involved ROC surfaces was extensively studied in Bantis and Feng (2018) [26]. The construction of joint confidence regions for the optimal TCF of ROC surfaces and hypersurfaces has been studied in-depth in Bantis et al. (2017) [15] and in Shi and Bantis (2022) [241]. Alternative cut-offs for the three class case and the k-class case have also been discussed in Hua and Tian (2020) [128] and in Feng and Tian (2022) [86]. Other advanced ROC surface analysis methods are described in Nakas and Reiser (2018) [189] and involve the works by Yin et al. (2018) [300], Inácio de Carvalho and Brunscam (2018) [132], Xiong et al. (2018) [292], and Zhang and Alonzo (2018) [304].

Further theoretical properties of the ROC surface and ROC hypersurface have also been studied in the literature [75–77, 81, 111–115, 229, 236, 240], while developments on the ROC umbrella have also appeared [85, 92].

5.9 Exercises

5.1 Calculate the VUS for the MoCA test using the Parkinson disease dataset of Section 1.4.4.

5.2 Compare the MoCA test with MMSE using both the VUS and the ROC surface directly under the trinormal model assumption using the `trinROC` package in `R`.

5.3 Estimate J_3 in the example of Section 5.7.1 using Equation (5.14).

5.4 Explore the changes in the estimation of the optimal cut-off points via J_3 for different weights in the importance of the different TCFs.

6

ROC Regression

CONTENTS

6.1 Regression Models for ROC Analysis 138
6.1.1 Parametric Methods 139
6.1.1.1 Ordinal categorical markers 139
6.1.1.2 Continuous markers 139
6.1.1.3 Computations 140
6.1.2 Semi-parametric Methods 141
6.1.2.1 Location-scale models 141
6.1.2.2 Cox regression models 142
6.1.3 Further reading 143
6.2 Optimal Prediction with Combinations of Markers 144
6.2.1 Prediction using machine learning techniques 145
6.2.2 Prediction using the binormal model 146
6.2.3 Biomarker combinations maximizing the Youden index 148
6.2.4 ROC curve evaluation after logistic regression 150
6.3 ROC Curve Analysis in Complex Designs 153
6.3.1 Analysis of correlated ordinal categorical data 153
6.3.2 Hierarchical ROC analysis 154
6.3.3 Jackknife and Bootstrap Methods 154
6.3.4 Sample size considerations 155
6.4 Time-dependent ROC Analysis 156
6.4.1 Definitions of time-dependent sensitivity and specificity 156
6.4.2 Estimation 157
6.4.3 Cumulative/dynamic 157
6.4.4 Incident/static 158
6.4.5 Incident/dynamic 159
6.5 Exercises 159

DOI: 10.1201/9780429170140-6

6.1 Regression Models for ROC Analysis

Variations in diagnostic performance have been reported for many types of diagnostic tests. For example, the DMIST trial, which compared the diagnostic accuracy of digital and film mammography in a screening population, reported that the estimated AUC (SE) for women under the age of 50 was 0.84 (0.03) for digital mammography and 0.69 (0.05) for film mammography. However, for the entire cohort of women in the study, the AUC estimates were 0.78 (0.02) and 0.74 (0.02), respectively [211]. Also, for women of age ≥ 65 years, the estimated AUC was 0.82 for those with mammographically dense breasts and 0.71 for those with mammographically nondense breasts [212]. Data from a reader study in which several radiologists interpreted a set of DMIST scans are summarized in Table 1.5.

Regression modeling provides an efficient way of examining variations in diagnostic performance. In addition, such models can be used to derive *adjusted* ROC curves. Insofar as the interpretation of adjusted curves and corresponding summary measures is heavily dependent on the modeling assumptions, the reporting and use of adjusted curves in practice needs to be done with considerable care.

A general class of regression models for tests or markers with ordinal categorical values was introduced in Chapter 3, Equation (3.4). In particular, if the marker Y takes values $1, 2, 3, ...C$, the general ordinal regression model has the form

$$P(Y_i \leq c|Z_i) = F(\frac{\theta_c - \alpha Z_i}{exp(\beta Z_i)}),$$

for $c = 1, ..., (C-1)$. Here Y_i denotes the marker value and Z_i denotes a vector of covariates on the i-th case, F denotes a cdf used to define the link function, α is called a *location parameter vector*, and β is called the *scale parameter vector*. Note that for $c = C$ the cumulative response probability is equal to 1. The use of ordinal regression models for a single and multiple markers was originally discussed in Tosteson and Begg (1988) [265] and Toledano and Gatsonis (1995) [262].

Regression models for markers taking continuous values have been constructed by modeling S_1 and S_2 as functions of the available covariates. Under a notation of $S_{1,Z}$ and $S_{2,Z}$ which implies the survival function of the biomarker scores given the covariate Z, the ROC curve model can be written as

$$ROC(t|Z) = S_{2,Z}(S_{1,Z}^{-1}(t)). \tag{6.1}$$

There are several methods discussed in the literature in how to accommodate Z [21, 45, 203, 204, 262, 263, 265, 314].

In this section, we present parametric, nonparametric, and semi-parametric approaches for the construction of the ROC curve and the estimation of the corresponding AUC given covariate information.

6.1.1 Parametric Methods

6.1.1.1 Ordinal categorical markers

We return now to the ordinal regression model with a covariate vector $Z = (D, Z_2, ...Z_k)$, where D denotes the binary indicator of the presence or absence of the target condition ("disease status"). Other components may include characteristics of the case and the test as well as interactions of these variables with disease status. For example, in the mammography study mentioned above, the response variable had seven possible categories ranging from "definitely not malignant" to "definitely malignant".

A model examining mammographic breast density as a factor related to the diagnostic accuracy would use $Z_i = (D_i, X_{1i}, D_i \times X_{1i})$ where D_i takes the value 1 if cancer is present in the i-th case and -1 if not, and X_{1i} takes the value 1 is the case has mammographically dense breasts and -1 if not. Note that the model can also accommodate studies in which density is measured on an ordinal categorical or continuous scale. If, for simplicity of the presentation, we assume no scale parameters (that is $\beta = 0$) and a Gaussian link, then $P(Y \leq c|Z) = \Phi(\theta_c - \alpha_1 D - \alpha_2 X - \alpha_3 D \cdot X)$. The last equation can be used to derive estimates of the ROC curve for cases in the two categories of density status.

We note here that researchers may also use the equation for deriving a single ROC curve that is "adjusted" for density. Because there is no consensus on the reference group for this adjustment, the analyst would need to define it precisely and also to justify the choice of reference group.

The ordinal regression approach can accommodate a variety of parametric shapes for the ROC curves and allows principled exploration of the effects of covariates, including the assessment of model fit, the handling of missing data, and the analysis of correlated responses [262, 263, 265].

6.1.1.2 Continuous markers

In the case of continuous valued markers, a similar approach begins with specifying a linear model for the marker X of the form [204]:

$$X_i = \beta_0 + \beta_1 D_i + \beta_2 Z_i + \beta_3 Z_i \times D_i + \sigma \cdot \epsilon, \tag{6.2}$$

where the error ϵ follows a standard normal distribution $N(0, 1)$, and σ is σ_1 for a non-diseased case and σ_2 for a diseased case. Note that the model assumes a different variance of the biomarker scores for the non-diseased and the diseased cases.

Under this parametrization, the ROC model can be written in the form of a binormal ROC curve as follows:

$$ROC(t) = \Phi\left(\frac{\beta_1}{\sigma_1} + \frac{\beta_3}{\sigma_2} Z + \frac{\sigma_1}{\sigma_2} \Phi^{-1}(1 - t)\right). \tag{6.3}$$

As in the case of the ordinal regression model, the covariate Z would have an effect on the ROC curve only when the interaction term has a non-zero coefficient (that is, $\beta_3 \neq 0$).

A more general form of the above parameterization is given by:

$$X_i = \mu(D_i, Z_i) + \sigma(D_i, Z_i)\epsilon,$$

which implies an ROC model of the form:

$$ROC_Z(t) = S_1\left(-a(Z) + b(Z)S_1^{-1}(t)\right), \tag{6.4}$$

with $a(Z) = \frac{(\mu(2,Z)-\mu(1,Z))}{\sigma(2,Z)}$, $b(Z) = \frac{\sigma(1,Z)}{\sigma(2,Z)}$.

The use of the above heteroscedastic linear regression models is also described in Zhou et al. (2011) [314] and are referred to as indirect strategies since they focus on modeling the marker scores as opposed to modeling the ROC directly given the covariates.

The above methods for performing a regression analysis of the ROC curve via modeling of the relation of the marker to covariates provide a transparent approach to this analysis. The face validity of assumptions about the relation of the covariates to the marker can be assessed on the basis of subject matter information in each case.

6.1.1.3 Computations

`Stata` has readily available functions and procedures for the implementation of a very wide range of ROC regression approaches. The documentations of `rocreg`, `rocreg postestimation`, and `rocregplot` offer a thorough overview of these models. An illustration of the use of these procedures in `Stata` using the pancreatic cancer data of Section 1.4.3 follows. In order to keep things simple, we exclude the pancreatic cancer group and focus on the separation between pancreatitis patients and otherwise healthy subjects for illustrative purposes only. We assess the accuracy of marker A1GL and the effect of ALB and CA19-9 on the corresponding ROC curve assessing the diagnostic accuracy of A1GL on the separation of diseased versus non-diseased subjects (where disease is pancreatitis for this simple example).

```
. gen true=group!=2
. quietly rocreg true a1gl, probit roccov(ca199 alb) bsave(pncrtest)

. set obs 70
number of observations (_N) was 67, now 70

. quietly replace alb = 40 in 67/70
. quietly replace ca199 = 10 in 67
. quietly replace ca199 = 30 in 68
. quietly replace ca199 = 50 in 69
. quietly replace ca199 = 70 in 70
```

```
. predict predAUC in 67/70, auc se(seAUC) bfile(pncrtest)

. list ca199 predAUC seAUC in 67/70

     +-----------------------------+
     | ca199    predAUC      seAUC |
     |-----------------------------|
 67. |    10   .7906489   .1098204 |
 68. |    30   .8209896   .0969945 |
 69. |    50   .8484037   .1011457 |
 70. |    70   .8728733   .1228208 |
     +-----------------------------+

. rocregplot, at1(ca199=10, alb=40) at2(ca199=50, alb=40)

* rocreg true a1gl, probit
* rocregplot
```

Using the model we obtain an estimated value of AUC for ALB=40 and a range of CA19-9 values, i.e. 10, 30, 50, 70. We observe that the diagnostic accuracy of A1GL increases at higher values of CA19-9 for a constant ALB measurement. Results are illustrated in Figure 6.1. Note that the AUC for A1GL with the use of the binormal model without covariate adjustment is equal to 0.800 with 95% CI:$(0.646, 0.905)$. Thorough assessment of a novel diagnostic marker can be a laborious task and it must be considered as such.

6.1.2 Semi-parametric Methods

Semi-parametric models for the relation of the marker to covariates have been proposed as building blocks of a regression analysis of the ROC curve. In particular, the proposals include the use of location-scale modeling [45, 203] and the use of Cox regression modeling of the marker [21].

6.1.2.1 Location-scale models

A model of this type is based on Equation (6.4) with the distribution of S_1 and the distribution of ϵ left unspecified. Quasi-likelihood can be used to solve the following estimating equation:

$$\sum\left(\left(\frac{\partial\mu(D,Z)}{\partial\beta}\right)\left(\frac{X-\mu_{D,Z}}{\sigma(D,Z)}\right)\right)=0, \tag{6.5}$$

where $\sigma(i,Z)=(\frac{1}{n_i}\sum(X_i-\mu(i,Z))^2)^{\frac{1}{2}}$, with $i=1,2$.

The empirical estimator, $\hat{S}_1$, can be used, with the corresponding ROC curve model written as [203]:

$$R\hat{O}C_Z(t)=\hat{S}_1\left(\frac{\mu(1,Z)-\mu(2,Z)}{\sigma(2,Z)}+\frac{\sigma(1,Z)}{\sigma(2,Z)}S_1^{-1}(t)\right). \tag{6.6}$$

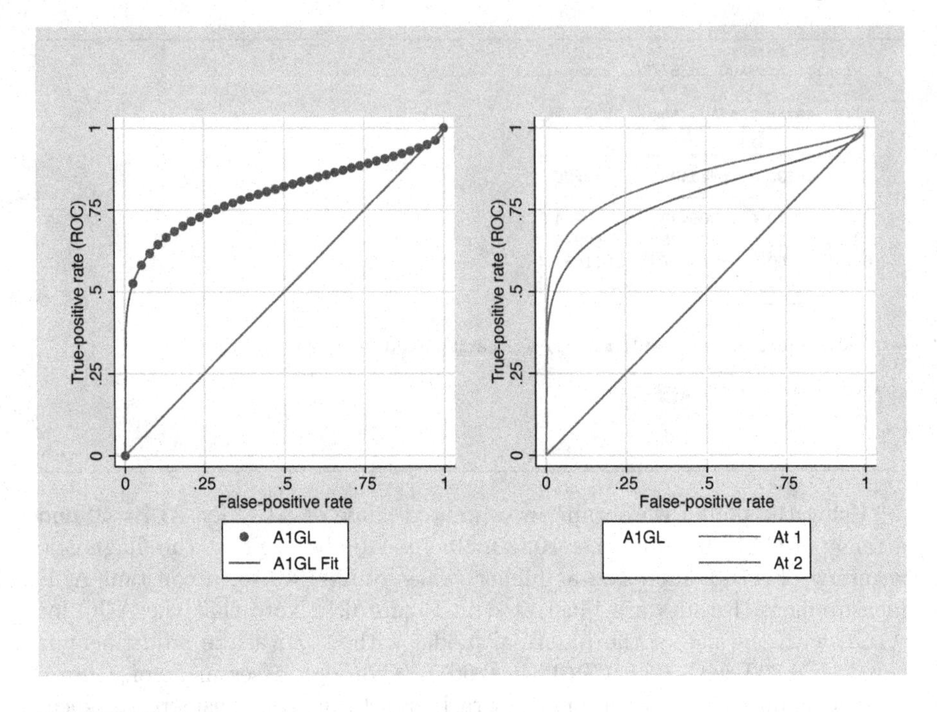

FIGURE 6.1
ROC curve for the marker A1GL, taking the effect of ALB, CA19-9 into account (right panel) for ALB=40 and CA19-9=10 (At1) and for ALB=40 and CA19-9=50 (At2). The ROC curve for A1GL only is also shown (left panel).

A more elaborate semi-parametric formulation is given by:

$$ROC_Z(t) = g\left(\beta' z + H(t)\right), \tag{6.7}$$

where $g(\cdot)$ is a link function as before, and $H(\cdot)$ is an unknown monotonically increasing function. For the technical details of estimation and inference, we refer the interested reader to the works of Cai (2004) [45] and Ghosh (2007) [95].

6.1.2.2 Cox regression models

A semi-parametric ROC regression model can be built using Cox regression [21]. The survival functions of the biomarker scores are estimated from the equation:

$$S(x|Z, D) = S_{base}(x)^{exp(\beta_1 Z + \beta_2 I(D=2))}, \tag{6.8}$$

where $I(A)$ is the indicator function of A and $S_{base}(x)$ is the baseline survival function for the marker scores. Such a formulation implies that for non-diseased cases ($D = 1$),

$$P(X > x|Z, D = 1) = S_{base}(x)^{exp(\beta_1 Z)},$$

and for diseased cases ($D = 2$) this yields,

$$P(X > x|Z, D = 2) = S_{base}(x)^{exp(\beta_1 Z + \beta_2)}.$$

As a result:

$$\frac{S(x|Z, D = 2)}{S(x|Z, D = 1)} = \frac{P(X > x|Z, D = 2)}{P(X > x|Z, D = 1)} = \frac{S_{base}(x)^{exp(\beta_1 Z + \beta_2)}}{S_{base}(x)^{exp(\beta_1 Z)}}$$

$$= S_{base}(x)^{\frac{[exp(\beta_1 Z)]}{[exp(\beta_2)-1]^{-1}}}.$$

Note that, for a given Z, the ratio of the cumulative distribution function of the biomarker scores for the diseased group over the non-diseased is also > 0. Also, if

$$S_{base}(x)^{[exp(\beta_1 Z)][exp(\beta_2)-1]} < 1,$$

then,

$$\frac{1 - F(x|Z, D = 2)}{1 - F(x|Z, D = 1)} < 1 \Rightarrow F(x|Z, D = 2) > F(x|Z, D = 1)$$

and the result is analogous if we consider the case where the left-hand side is > 1. That is, for any x, the distributions of the two groups are stochastically ordered.

When implementing two separate Cox models, one for the non-diseased and one for the diseased, we gain some additional flexibility since we allow the covariates to have a different effect on the non-diseased and diseased groups. Employing a unified Cox model that involves the disease status as a covariate has the benefit of an increased power, but comes at the cost of such flexibility (of questionable usefulness, since the disease status will be unknown in a predictive framework).

A complication regarding the interpretation of this model involves the addition of more covariates. Each new covariate in Z implies that we are willing to assume a more strict condition on the type of stochastic ordering. Regarding the baseline function, it can be left completely unspecified or restricted splines could be used instead such as the HCNS method discussed in Bantis et al. (2012) [21]. The implementation of the HCNS can be done through a MATLAB package available for download at `www.leobantis.net` and discussed in detail in Bantis et al. (2020) [23].

6.1.3 Further reading

Brumback et al. (2006) [43] discuss a GLM-based technique to adjust the AUC for covariates. Other strategies for accommodating covariates in an ROC framework have been more recently suggested. A semi-parametric linear regression framework was proposed by Zhang and Huang (2005) [305] which allows the estimate of the sensitivity at a given specificity to vary based on the covariates. Rodriguez-Alvarez et al. (2011) [224] discuss the accommodation of the covariate effects in a nonparametric fashion and further discuss bootstrap based inference in Rodriguez-Alvarez et al. (2018) [225]. Cox-based models in combination with constrained cubic splines are discussed in Bantis et al. (2012) [21] in an ROC surface setting. A Dirichlet-dependent, nonparametric bayesian approach is discussed by Inácio de Carvalho et al. (2013) [133]. Therein, the authors further discuss exact posterior inference. Even though all these methods can be used to also calculate a covariate-adjusted AUC, there are also methods that focus mainly on the AUC such as the one presented by Yao et al. (2009) [298] whose methods fall under the umbrella of methods in Pepe (1998) [203] and are in turn more general than the methods presented in Faraggi (2003) [83] and in Schisterman et al. (2004) [233].

The interested reader is referred to the article by To et al. (2022) [259] for VUS estimation in the presence of covariates. Semi-parametric estimation of the ROC surface was studied by Li and Zhou (2009) [150] generalizing the results of the two-class case in Hsieh and Turnbull (1996) [127], and by Nze Ossima et al. (2013) [194] generalizing the results of the two-class case in Gönen and Heller (2010) [96]. The estimation of the ROC surface of a diagnostic marker with continuous measurements given covariate information has been considered in Li et al. (2012) [151].

6.2 Optimal Prediction with Combinations of Markers

In practice, a single marker is rarely used to diagnose disease or make a prognosis for an outcome. A group of markers might be used and baseline characteristics might also be taken into account.

High-throughput technologies that can simultaneously assay a large number of markers using minimal resources especially in terms of biospecimens/blood have contributed toward the development of techniques that combine diagnostic information in a more straightforward way than the framework described in the previous section. Once the most promising markers have been filtered out of a, usually, large list of candidates, investigators may be interested in constructing a combination of those that can complement each other and refine, while simplifying in practice, the diagnostic task. Complementing biomarkers may be focusing/detecting different features that are associated with the disease under study.

A combination of biomarkers, possibly including other baseline characteristics, will be considered to be "optimal" if it results in an ROC curve that is "better" than any other ROC curve derived from a different combination of the same biomarkers. The term "better" refers to a comparison measure, such as the AUC, pAUC, J, or any other ROC-related criterion. As a result, the "optimal" combination will have the higher AUC among all other combinations of the same markers if the AUC is the target measure, or stated more formally, objective function.

Normal linear combinations maximizing the AUC have been studied by Su and Liu (1993) [254]. Further developments followed by several authors (e.g. [78,169,219] among others), while distribution-free approaches for linear combinations have also been studied (e.g. [161, 205] among others). Linear combinations using J as the objective function were studied in Yin and Tian (2014) [301]. Other textbooks describing these approaches include Zou et al. (2012) [318] and Matsui et al. (2015) [165].

Yan et al. (2018) [295] present a framework to maximize the pAUC for a given pre-determined FPR range of interest $(a - b)$. It is obvious that this framework includes the AUC when one considers $a = 0$ and $b = 1$. As in the previous sections, we will consider both parametric and nonparametric options. Below we discuss the parametric case of multivariate normality as well as nonparametric methods to maximize AUC, or pAUC, when deriving a linear combination of markers.

6.2.1 Prediction using machine learning techniques

From a machine learning perspective, a common goal is to build an ensemble of weak prediction models, usually decision trees, through extreme gradient boosting methodology. An optimal combination of markers is produced, which results in an optimal prediction model, in the sense that the maximum possible AUC is achieved.

An illustration on the use of this approach in R using the pancreatic cancer data of Section 1.4.3 is as follows.

```
pankr13b<-read.csv(file.choose())
pankr13b<-pankr13b[pankr13b$X...Group!=1,]

library(xgboost)
grouping<-pankr13b$X...Group!=2
group2Bd <- as.numeric(grouping)
kmarkers<-as.matrix(cbind(pankr13b$A1GL,pankr13b$ALB,pankr13b$CA199))

xmarkcomb <- xgboost(data = kmarkers, label = group2Bd,
max.depth = 5, eta = 0.3, nrounds=10, nthread = 10,
objective = "binary:logistic", eval_metric = 'auc')
importance_mtrx=xgb.importance(feature_names=c("a1gl","alb","ca199"),
model = xmarkcomb)
#importance_mtrx
```

```
cv.combmark <- xgb.cv(data = kmarkers, nfold = 10, max.depth = 5,
eta = 0.3, nthread = 10, nrounds=10, label = group2Bd,
verbose = FALSE, objective = 'binary:logistic',
eval_metric = 'auc', prediction = T)

library(pROC)
xgbrocs<-roc(response = group2Bd,
             predictor = cv.combmark$pred,
             levels=c(0, 1))
xgbrocs
plot.roc(xgbrocs, legacy.axes=TRUE)

plot.roc(smooth(xgbrocs), legacy.axes=TRUE)

ci.sp.obj <- ci.sp(smooth(xgbrocs), sensitivities=seq(0, 1, .01),
boot.n=250)
plot(smooth(xgbrocs), legacy.axes=TRUE) # restart a new plot
plot(ci.sp.obj, type="shape", col="aquamarine1", legacy.axes=TRUE)
```

The estimated AUC for prediction is 0.8433, while the AUC from the testing sample was 0.992. The former along with corresponding confidence intervals is presented in Figure 6.2.

6.2.2 Prediction using the binormal model

In this section, we discuss optimal prediction using a combination of continuous markers under the normality assumption. We consider one multivariate normal distribution for the diseased group $\boldsymbol{X}_2$ and another for the non-diseased group $\boldsymbol{X}_1$, i.e., $\boldsymbol{X}_2 \sim MVN(\boldsymbol{\mu}_2, \boldsymbol{\Sigma}_2)$ and $\boldsymbol{X}_1 \sim MVN(\boldsymbol{\mu}_1, \boldsymbol{\Sigma}_1)$, where $\boldsymbol{\mu}_2$ and $\boldsymbol{\mu}_1$ are the mean vectors for the disease and non-disease groups, respectively; and $\boldsymbol{\Sigma}_2$ and $\boldsymbol{\Sigma}_1$ are the $m \times m$ covariance matrices for the diseased and non-diseased groups, respectively. Let $\boldsymbol{\beta} = (\beta_1, \beta_2, \ldots, \beta_m)$ be the vector of coefficients based on which we can construct a linear combination of m biomarkers. It follows that $\boldsymbol{W}_2$ and $\boldsymbol{W}_1$, the *combined scores* that correspond to diseased and non-diseased groups, follow univariate normal distributions:

$$\boldsymbol{W}_2 = \boldsymbol{\beta}^T \boldsymbol{X}_2 \sim N(\mu_{\boldsymbol{W}_2}, \sigma^2_{\boldsymbol{W}_2}),\ \boldsymbol{W}_1 = \boldsymbol{\beta}^T \boldsymbol{X}_1 \sim N(\mu_{\boldsymbol{W}_1}, \sigma^2_{\boldsymbol{W}_1}),$$

where their means are given by $\mu_{\boldsymbol{W}_2} = \boldsymbol{\beta}^T \boldsymbol{\mu}_2$ and $\mu_{\boldsymbol{W}_1} = \boldsymbol{\beta}^T \boldsymbol{\mu}_1$ and the variances of the combined scores are $\sigma^2_{\boldsymbol{W}_2} = \boldsymbol{\beta}^T \boldsymbol{\mu}_2 \boldsymbol{\beta}$ and $\sigma^2_{\boldsymbol{W}_1} = \boldsymbol{\beta}^T \boldsymbol{\mu}_1 \boldsymbol{\beta}$ respectively.

As previously discussed, it may be the case that clinical interest lies on a specific range of FPR values. For example, if we are dealing with early

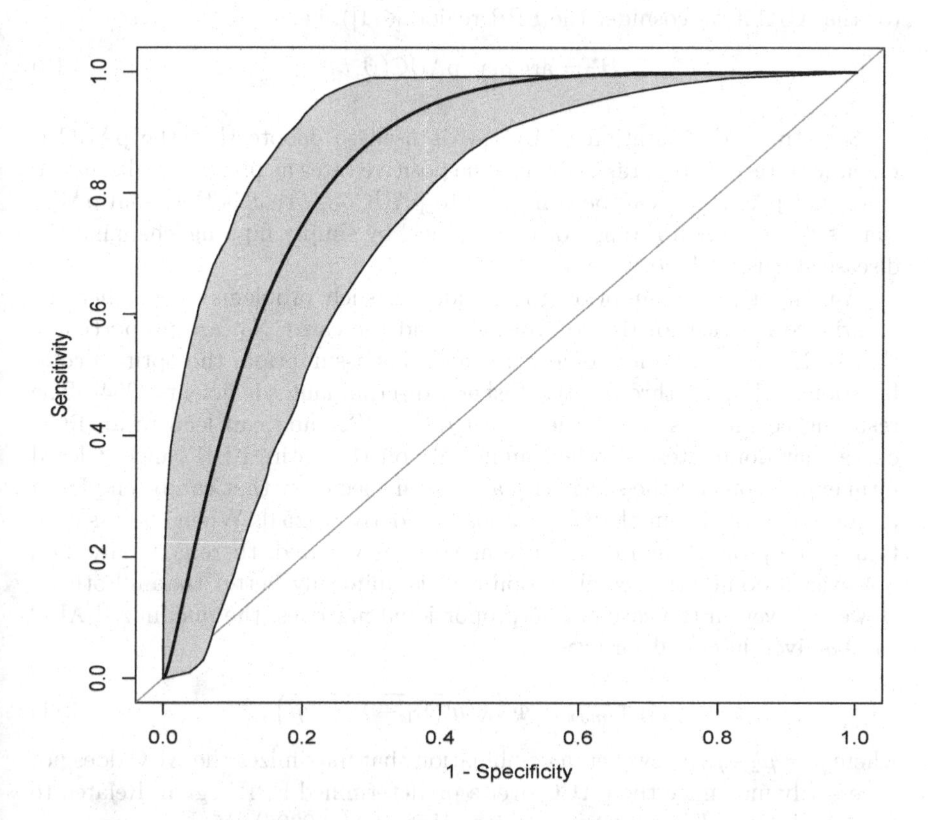

FIGURE 6.2
Combination of markers A1GL, ALB, CA19-9 to an overall score for the pancreatic cancer data, using only the healthy and pancreatitis groups for illustration. ROC curve produced via extreme gradient boosting.

detection it is usually of interest to focus on very low FPR values so that we spare healthy individuals from unnecessary invasive follow-ups. On the other hand, if we are dealing with a disease that is at an advanced stage, we are more interested in forcing high TPR rates. In either scenario, we can formulate the problem without loss of generality on a clinically relevant FPR region $[0, t_0]$. The pAUC of the combined scores is defined as

$$\text{pAUC}(\boldsymbol{\beta}, t_0) = \int_0^{t_0} \text{ROC}(t)dt = \int_0^{t_0} \Phi\left(\frac{\mu_{\boldsymbol{W}_2} - \mu_{\boldsymbol{W}_1} + \sigma_{\boldsymbol{W}_2}\Phi^{-1}(t)}{\sigma_{\boldsymbol{W}_2}}\right) dt \tag{6.9}$$

where Φ is the cumulative distribution function of the standard normal distribution. Note that the AUC is simply a special case of the pAUC that corresponds to selecting $[0, 1]$ instead of $[0, t_0]$. The goal is to find the optimal linear coefficients $\boldsymbol{\beta}^*$ that maximized the pAUC over the FPR region $[0, t_0]$

(or the AUC if we cosnider the FPR region $[0,1]$), i.e.,

$$\boldsymbol{\beta}^* = \arg\max_{\boldsymbol{\beta}} \mathrm{pAUC}(\boldsymbol{\beta}, t_0). \tag{6.10}$$

Sometimes the notation $\mathrm{pAUC}_{\mathrm{TPR}}$ is used to denote that the pAUC is taken with respect to a range of the true positive rates as previously discussed. Note that $\mathrm{pAUC}_{\mathrm{TPR}}$ can be converted to $\mathrm{pAUC}_{\mathrm{FPR}}$, that is the usual pAUC that is defined upon a range of FPR values, by simply flipping/changing the disease status of the original data.

An important assumption to consider in such problems is whether the covariance matrices of the controls, Σ_1, and the cases, Σ_2, are proportional, that is, $\Sigma_2 = \sigma^2 \times \Sigma_1$ for some σ^2. Under this assumption, the optimal combination is derived through the Fisher's discriminant coefficients [254]. The resulting coefficients are of the form $(\mu_1 - \mu_2)'\Sigma_1$ and can lead to an ROC curve that dominates all others uniformly on the entire FPR range. Closed form expressions for the sensitivity at a given specificity that can be employed to construct the optimal ROC can also be derived [254]. When the assumption of the proportional covariance matrices is violated, there generally does not exist a dominating combination that is uniformly better than all others. However, even in the case of non-proportional matrices, the maximized AUC can be given in closed form:

$$AUC_{max} = \Phi\left(\sqrt{\mu'(\Sigma_1 + \Sigma_2)^{-1}\mu}\right), \tag{6.11}$$

where $\mu = \mu_2 - \mu_1$. However, a combination that maximizes the AUC does not necessarily maximize the pAUC over a predetermined FPR region. Related to favoring high or low specificity regions, Liu et al. (2006) [153] discuss linear combinations that dominate all others. However, their approach cannot be pre-specified to operate under a desired predetermined region of FPRs. Thus, it cannot guarantee a maximized pAUC within a clinically relevant region of interest.

A kernel-based approach through the usual kernel density estimator has been described in Yan et al. (2018) [295] as a nonparametric analog to the process described above. A `Matlab` function named `maxpauckernall.m` for the relevant implementation can be found at `www.leobantis.net`. It requires a matrix M where each of its columns reflects one marker (and each row represents one individual), the disease status, and an FPR range on which the pAUC is to be optimized. Figure 6.3 provides a relevant illustration.

6.2.3 Biomarker combinations maximizing the Youden index

Combining biomarkers based on the maximum of the Youden index is an alternative way of creating scores that encompass information of a set of markers. A nonparametric min-max approach that linearly combines the minimum and the maximum scores of m biomarkers has been described in the literature [155]. In what follows, a step wise approach is described [301] which

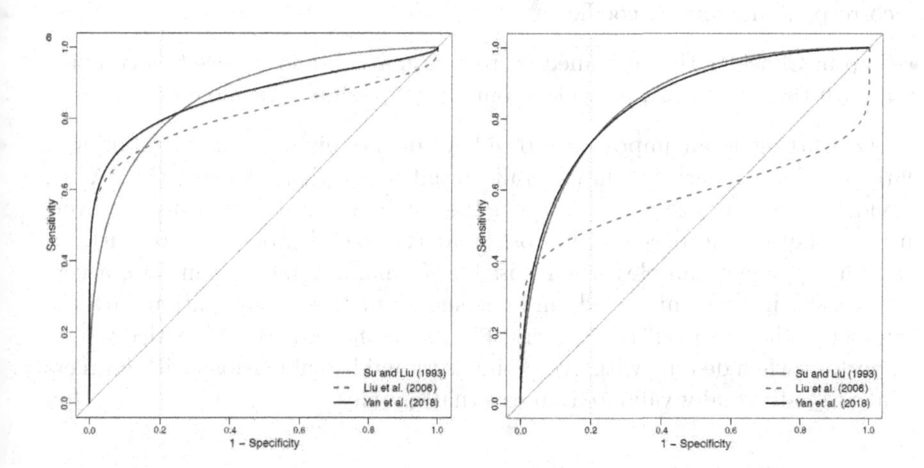

FIGURE 6.3
Example of a combination of two markers where both groups are normally distributed with non-proportional covariance matrices and underlying parameters. Left: $\mu_2 = (3,3)$, $\mu_1 = (0,0)$, $\sigma_2 = (3,2)$, $\sigma_1 = (1,2)$. The underlying correlation is 0.5. Su and Liu's approach exhibit the largest AUC; however, the largest pAUC over the region of interest (here is $FPR = [0, 0.2]$) is attained by the Yan et al. method [295]. Right: $\mu_2 = (1,3)$, $\mu_1 = (0,0)$.

outperforms the min-max approach and thus we will only focus on the latter. The corresponding algorithm consists of the following steps:

- Step 1: Derive the empirical estimate of the maximum of the Youden index for each one of the biomarkers to be combined.
- Step 2: Order the m biomarkers based on their maximized Youden indices from the largest to the smallest. Denote these values for the diseased group with $x_{2i} = (x_{2i,(p)}, x_{2i,(p-1)}, \ldots, x_{2i,(1)})'$ and for the non-diseased as $x_{1i} = (x_{1i,(p)}, x_{1i,(p-1)}, \ldots, x_{1i,(1)})'$.
- Step 3: Combine the first two biomarkers by considering the first as an anchor (forcing its coefficient equal to 1) and scan for the coefficient of the second in the interval [-1, 1] with 210 equally spaced points.
- Step 4: Combine the first two biomarkers by considering the second as an anchor and scan for the coefficient of the second in the interval [-1, 1] with 210 equally spaces points.

- Step 5: Determine which of two previous steps yields a larger maximum of the respective Youden index and combine them accordingly with the corresponding derived coefficient.
- Step 6: Consider the combined score as a marker, and proceed to combine it with the next (third in rank) biomarker in a similar fashion, etc.

Overfitting is an important consideration in this context. Combining a large number of markers will generally result in a higher AUC (or the pAUC, Youden index etc). To assess whether the combination is not subject to overfitting, one could proceed with cross-validation-based procedures or with totally independent samples when possible. Combining more than 10 markers is generally not recommended, and one should proceed with caution with the number of the contributing markers [129]. A further aspect in practice that is important when dealing with overfitting is to build combinations with markers that are individually validated on external samples.

6.2.4 ROC curve evaluation after logistic regression

A straightforward, yet non-optimal, method to proceed with marker combinations is the use of the binary logistic regression model. The linear predictor term of the logistic regression model can serve as a diagnostic/prognostic score. That is, model the disease status with the biomarker scores, or any other baseline characteristic of interest, as covariates:

$$logit(P(D=2))/(1-P(D=2))) = \beta_0+\beta_1 \cdot X_1+\beta_2 \cdot X_2+\ldots+\beta_p \cdot X_k, \quad (6.12)$$

where $X_1, X_2, \ldots, X_k$ is a set of biomarkers and baseline characteristics of interest. Their combined effect on the presence of the target condition is modelled, typically, using maximum likelihood methodology.

Fitting such a model can be done through any standard statistical software using either the logit or the probit link function since the target condition status is binary. Then, one may simply extract the linear term of the model (that can either include or exclude the intercept of the model) and consider the combined score as a pseudoscore representing the diagnostic profile of any given individual. This strategy has been extensively used in the literature and has been discussed in several books on machine learning, statistical modeling, and relevant articles (e.g. [147,165,217]).

An illustration of the use of this approach in `R` using the pancreatic cancer data once again follows. In order to keep things consistent, we exclude the pancreatic cancer group and focus on the separation between pancreatitis patients and otherwise healthy subjects. We combine markers A1GL, ALB, CA19-9 using a binary logistic regression model, where the target condition is pancreatitis. In particular, after fitting the binary logistic regression model that considers the disease status as the response and the biomarkers as covariates, we focus solely on its linear term. Using the linear term, we can create a combined score (or pseudoscore) that we then consider as a combined marker itself. The individual ROCs along with the ROC of the pseudoscore are presented in Figure 6.4.

```
pankr13<-read.csv(file.choose())
#download from http://dx.doi.org/10.13140/RG.2.2.20621.08160
pankr13<-pankr13[pankr13$Group!=1,]
library(pROC)
#roc(Group~A1GL,pankr13, auc=T, ci=T)
#roc(Group~CA199,pankr13, auc=T, ci=T)
#roc(Group~ALB,pankr13, auc=T, ci=T)

plot(roc(Group~A1GL,pankr13, auc=T, ci=T), lty=2)
par(new=T)
plot(roc(Group~ALB,pankr13, auc=T, ci=T), lty=3)
par(new=T)
plot(roc(Group~CA199,pankr13, auc=T, ci=T), lty=4)
par(new=T)

grouping<-pankr13$Group!=2
mod <- glm(grouping ~ pankr13$A1GL + pankr13$ALB +
             pankr13$CA199, family="binomial")
beta1 <- mod$coefficients[[2]]
beta2 <- mod$coefficients[[3]]
beta3 <- mod$coefficients[[4]]

pseudoscores<- pankr13$A1GL*beta1+pankr13$ALB*beta2+
  pankr13$CA199*beta3

#roc(pankr13$Group~pseudoscores, auc=T, ci=T)
plot(roc(pankr13$Group~pseudoscores, auc=T, ci=T), lty=1)

legend(0.4, 0.3,
       legend=c("Pseudoscores", "A1GL", "ALB", "CA199"), lty=1:4)
c(beta1, beta2, beta3)        #display betas
```

```
## [1]  2.3829240 -0.2923280  0.1110465
```

The combined score results in an overall higher AUC equal to 0.872 (95% CI: 0.782, 0.962) compared to the individual AUCs. Specifically, for A1GL, AUC=0.785 (95% CI: 0.655, 0.916); for ALB, AUC= 0.803 (95% CI: 0.688, 0.918); for CA19-9, AUC=0.688 (95% CI: 0.551, 0.824). All three markers significantly separate between healthy subjects and pancreatitis cases; however, the combined score results in a higher AUC in absolute terms. Classical model building approaches can be used for the construction of the combined marker

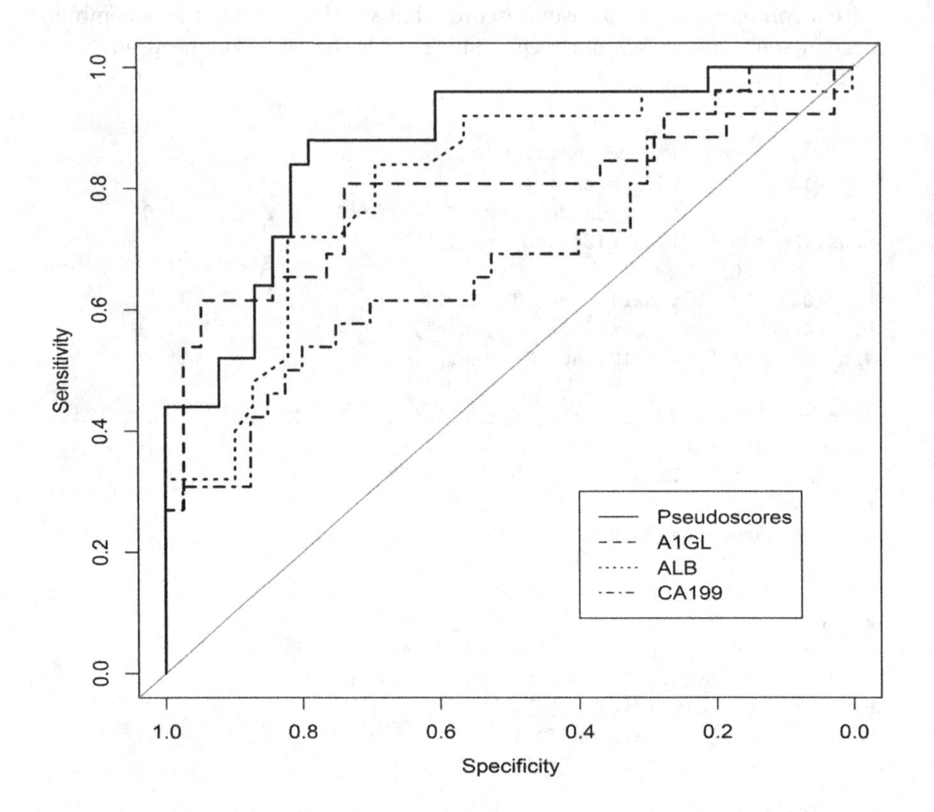

FIGURE 6.4
Combination of markers A1GL, ALB, CA19-9 to an overall score for the pancreatic cancer data, using only the healthy and pancreatitis groups for illustration. ROC curves corresponding to the individual markers and the overall score are shown.

(see e.g. Hosmer et al. (2013) [126]), while the added value of a biomarker to a set of biomarkers in a model can be assessed using methods outlined in Chapter 4 or via other ad hoc sophisticated approaches (such as Heller et al. (2017) [119]). A broad range of such approaches is summarized in Cook (2018) [56].

A drawback of the use of the binary logistic regression model as described above is that the estimation process for the pseudoscore is not accuracy based. Specifically, the logistic regression model is produced by maximizing a likelihood function rather than an accuracy/ROC-based measure and following such a strategy does not guarantee that there are no other linear combinations of the same markers that yield a larger AUC, which in turn implies a larger discriminatory capacity of the resulting combined marker (also referred to as a panel or a composite biomarker).

6.3 ROC Curve Analysis in Complex Designs

Correlated ROC data arise in many studies of diagnostic accuracy, primarily because participants are often assessed using more than one biomarker or imaging modality. In the case of imaging studies, scans may also be interpreted by multiple human readers or multiple AI software. We have already discussed the commonly used paired design for the comparison of markers in Chapter 4. In this design, each case (participant) is assessed using two markers and the design and analysis accounts for the correlation induced by the pairing. As can be seen from Section 4.2, the analytic methods can be readily extended to handle situations with multiple assessments per case. In this section, we provide an overview of methods for multiple correlated marker data and also discuss design considerations.

6.3.1 Analysis of correlated ordinal categorical data

A fixed effects analysis of correlated ROC data can be carried out using a generalization of the ordinal regression ROC model which was discussed in Section 3.1.1.2. The generalization employs generalized estimating equations (GEE) techniques to account for the correlation [262]. In particular, an ordinal regression model is used for each of the repeated responses (such as interpretations of the same scan by different readers or marker values obtained by different methods), but the parameters are allowed to vary between assessment occasions. Estimates of all parameters are obtained and a robust estimate of the covariance matrix is also generated, which takes into consideration the correlations that exist between the repeated readings for each subject.

The GEE model allows us to derive and compare ROC curves for each modality or marker and for each test interpreter. Estimates of areas under each ROC curve are unbiased even in small data sets. Standard errors of quantities, such as the difference in average area for each modality, are estimated appropriately for the readers in the sample and can be easily adjusted to allow generalization beyond the current reader sample.

In the case of studies in which multiple readers interpret scans for each modality, the GEE approach also allows construction of a *summary* ROC curve, e.g., for each modality, through averages of the parameters determining the individual ROC curves, e.g., for each reader [264]. We note that the GEE approach can also accommodate the presence of missing data in the ordinal categorical response (for example, when one of the readers has not interpreted a particular specimen) [263,290]. Alternatives to the GEE approach for analyzing multi-reader ROC data include the jackknife and bootstrap methods discussed in the next paragraphs [14,28,71], ANOVA modeling of areas under the curve or other ROC summary measures [195,256], a marginal model approach [250], and nonparametric methods [196,249].

6.3.2 Hierarchical ROC analysis

Hierarchical regression models can also be used to study variation in diagnostic performance across test interpreters, human or AI, and to account for correlations in multi-reader studies [93,134]. As an example, consider studies in which a number of readers interpret the same set of cases. Studies of this type are routinely conducted within multicenter trials to derive estimates of both the center and the dispersion of the diagnostic performance of radiologists and to assess possible contributing factors.

From a design viewpoint, key questions include the selection of the numbers of readers and cases, as well as the pattern of readings. From an analysis viewpoint, key issues include the formulation of appropriate models and the development of efficient computational algorithms and methods from assessing model fit.

The fundamental building block in the hierarchical regression model is the ordinal regression model described in Section 3.1.1.2. The following general class of hierarchical models can incorporate both patient- and reader-level covariates. If Y_{ik} is the response of reader i on case k, with case-level covariate vector $Z_k^{(2)}$ of length n_2, (always including indicator of true disease status), and reader-level covariate vector $Z_i^{(1)}$ of length n_1, the hierarchical model will have the following general structure:

Level I: Within-reader variation: $h^{-1}(P[Y_{ik} \leq j]) = \frac{\theta_{ij} - \alpha_i Z_k^{(2)}}{e^{\beta_i Z_k^{(2)}}}$.

Level II: Between-reader variation: The reader-specific ordinal regression coefficients are modeled as functions of variables representing reader characteristics plus error. For example, $\alpha_{i1} = \gamma_{10} + \gamma_{11} Z_{i1}^{(1)} + ... + \gamma_{1n_z} Z_{in_1}^{(1)} + \epsilon_{i1}$, and similarly for the scale parameters.

Level III: Vague but proper priors are assumed on the second-stage parameters.

A class of models of this form is discussed by Ishwaran and Gatsonis (2000) [134] and applied to data from two multi-reader, multi-modality studies. The models make it possible to develop estimates of the variability across readers (human or AI software) and estimates of the effects covariates, reflecting characteristics of the cases and characteristics of the readers.

6.3.3 Jackknife and Bootstrap Methods

This class of methods focuses on the analysis of a particular summary statistic of the ROC curve, such as the AUC, rather than the ROC curve itself. The jackknife method [71] derives a "pseudovalue" area for each case by removing that case from the data set and then estimating the area under the curve with the remaining cases (hence the "jackknife"). Those pseudovalue areas are then modeled via mixed effects ANOVA, where the random effects indicate components of variance that are of interest. Not all components of variance are identifiable without substantial replication, and this has implications for the design and analysis of *multiple reader, multiple modality studies* [70,226].

Estimation of the components of variance in the ANOVA model is of interest, because they indicate variability due to specific sources, such as the cases, readers, or modalities [226]. Beiden et al. (2000) [31] developed a multiple bootstrap approach for random effects ROC curve analysis that is more flexible than the original jackknife method. The added flexibility is gained because the variance components are estimated via the bootstrap of the jackknife pseudovalues, rather than fitting a mixed effects ANOVA model.

The `R` package `iMRMC` implements such methods, also detailed in Gallas et al. (2009) [91].

6.3.4 Sample size considerations

The computation of sample sizes of cases and readers in multi-reader, multi-case (MRMC) studies is generally considerably more complex than the methods discussed in Chapter 4. The mixed model approach [195,201] is often used in practice.

For a study in which each of J readers interpret scans taken on the same cases by one of I modalities, the mixed model for the estimated AUC of the jth reader interpreting scans from the ith modality form is

$$\hat{\theta}_{ij} = \mu + \alpha_i + \beta_j + (\alpha\beta)_{ij} + \epsilon_{ij}$$

where μ denotes the grand mean, α_i denotes the effect of modality i (fixed), β_j denotes the effect of reader j (random), $(\alpha\beta)$ denotes the reader by modality interaction (random), and ϵ_{ij} denotes the random error term. The random terms are assumed to be normally distributed with mean zero.

In the notation of the mixed model, the AUC of test i is $\theta_i = \mu + \alpha_i$. The test statistic for the hypothesis $H_0 : \theta_1 = \theta_2$, (that is, the AUC of the two tests is the same) follows an $F_{1,(J-1)}$ distribution under the null hypothesis. Sample size and power calculations require the non-central F distribution and its non-centrality parameter. In order to derive a value for the non-centrality parameter, the analyst would need to estimate several quantities, including the variance for readers σ^2_β, the variance for the reader by modality interaction $\sigma^2_{\alpha\beta}$, and the variance of the error term σ^2_ϵ. Equicovariance is typically assumed for the error terms, which means the analyst would only need to specify the covariance for three types of terms, $Cov(\epsilon_{ij}, \epsilon_{i'j'})$ when $i \neq i', j \neq j'$, or $i = i', j \neq j'$ or $i \neq i', j = j'$. Even with these simplifications, the derivation of the non-centrality parameter requires substantial information. The interested reader may consult Chapter 6 of Zhou et al. (2011) [314] and also Hillis and

Schartz (2018) [122]. The latter reference describes a software for computing sample sizes for MRMC designs which was further developed into the `R` package `MRMCaov`.

6.4 Time-dependent ROC Analysis

Many disease outcomes, such as overall survival or disease-free survival, are defined as time-to-event outcomes. The prediction of such outcomes is of great interest as already stated in Section 1.2.1. For example, as outlined in Heagerty et al. (2000) [116], the percent cells in the synthesis phase (S-phase) are correlated with survival. Other examples may refer to the levels of CD4 cell counts when dealing with HIV patients, the Framingham Risk Score which can be predictive of myocardial infarction and stroke etc. Hence, methods that can characterize the time-varying accuracy of a marker under a scope of dynamic decision-making have been developed. To evaluate a continuous or ordinal marker under a time-dependent setting, the notions of sensitivity and specificity need to be extended to accommodate dynamic information. This is achieved in a survival analysis context and an obvious implication is that censoring might occur. The approach proposed by Heagerty et al. (2000) [116] is discussed in the sequel. Packages `smoothROCtime` [66] and `ROCt` implement these procedures in `R`. An insightful application of such methods is given in Han et al. (2020) [102].

6.4.1 Definitions of time-dependent sensitivity and specificity

Consider that $\mathcal{T}_i$ is the failure time and that X_i refers to the marker value of individual i. Denote with C_i the censoring time variable. In a given application, we are not in position of observing all failure times. Instead, we only observe $Z_i = \min(\mathcal{T}_i, C_i)$ which is the follow-up time. In addition, we also have the information given by the censoring indicator $\delta_i = I(\mathcal{T}_i \leq C_i)$ that indicates whether a data point refers to a censored or a fully observed time. Cases and controls are defined through a counting process: $D(t) = 1$ if $\mathcal{T}_i < t$ and $D(t) = 0$ if $\mathcal{T}_i > t$. With $D(t) = 1$ we indicate that individual i experienced an event before time t. Since now the true disease status is time-dependent, the notions of both the sensitivity and specificity are analogously extended:

$$sensitivity(c, t) = P(X > c|D(t) = 2) \tag{6.13}$$

$$specificity(c, t) = P(X \leq c|D(t) = 1) \tag{6.14}$$

These definitions imply that for a given time point t and a given cut-off c, we obtain a pair of (sensitivity, specificity). That is, for a given time point

t, we can scan for all possible values of the cut-off and derive the *ROC* curve that corresponds to that particular time point t.

6.4.2 Estimation

Using Bayes theorem, we can derive:

$$P(X > c|D(t) = 2) = \frac{(1 - S(t|X > c))P(X > c)}{1 - S(t)} \quad (6.15)$$

$$P(X \leq c|D(t) = 1) = \frac{(S(t|X \leq c))P(X \leq c)}{S(t)} \quad (6.16)$$

where $S(t) = P(\mathcal{T} > t)$. A common nonparametric estimate of $S(t)$ is the well-known Kaplan-Meier (KM) estimator, which can take into account all data points including those that refer to censored time points. Using such an estimate for the survival function and the empirical estimate for the cdf of the marker X we obtain:

$$\hat{P}_{KM}(X > c|D(t) = 2) = \frac{1 - \hat{S}_{KM}(t|X > c)(1 - \hat{F}_X(c))}{1 - \hat{S}_{KM}(t)} \quad (6.17)$$

$$\hat{P}_{KM}(X > c|D(t) = 1) = \frac{\hat{S}_{KM}(t|X \leq c)\hat{F}_X(c)}{\hat{S}_{KM}(t)} \quad (6.18)$$

However, this estimator does not guarantee that the sensitivity (or specificity) is monotone [116]. The Kaplan–Meier estimates through Bayes theorem do not necessarily comply with the desired monotonicity because $\hat{P}(X > c, \mathcal{T} > t) = \hat{S}_{KM}(t|X_i > c)(1 - \hat{F}_X(c))$ may not provide a valid bivariate distribution estimate. However, a valid estimation of the aforementioned bivariate distribution function is given by Akritas (1994) [3] based on nearest neighbor estimation.

There are two distinct settings that refer to the aforementioned extensions of the sensitivity/specificity. The distinction is based on whether the cases are "incident cases", defined for $\mathcal{T}_i = t$, or "cumulative cases" that are defined for $\mathcal{T}_i \leq t$. The controls can be considered either as "static" that correspond to $\mathcal{T}_i > t^*$ for a pre-defined fixed t^* or "dynamic" defined for subjects for which $\mathcal{T}_i > t$.

6.4.3 Cumulative/dynamic

For this definition, we define the cumulative cases (C) as subjects who experience the event before time t and controls are defined by those who remain event-free beyond time t. If we denote with $\mathcal{T}$ the survival time and with s, the time point at case ascertainment which is often taken as 0 to refer to baseline. Thus, cases are those individuals who experience the event in (s, t). Controls are dynamic (D) and are those who are event free beyond t, i.e. $\mathcal{T}_i > t$. Based on this definition, the sensitivity and specificity at a cut-off c are defined as:

$$sensitivity^C(c,t) : P(X_i > c|\mathcal{T}_i \leq t) = TPR_t^C \tag{6.19}$$

$$specificity^D(c,t) : P(X_i \leq c|\mathcal{T}_i > t) = 1 - FPR_t^D \tag{6.20}$$

Using this definition, the fixed time t dichotomizes the sample in to cases and controls. Observe that a single individual that contributes as a control for $t < \mathcal{T}_i$, but at later times it contributes as a case. As in the our previously discussed settings, if we scan the cut-off c on the real line we obtain infinite pairs of sensitivity and specificity that if plotted on the plane form the time dependent ROC, more specifically:

$$ROC_t^{C/D}(p) = TPR_t^C((FPR_t^D)^{-1}(p)). \tag{6.21}$$

Hence, under this context, the area uder the ROC curve is given by:

$$AUC_t = \int_0^1 ROC_t^{C/D}(p)dp, \tag{6.22}$$

which by definition allows us to examine the trajectory of the AUC, which reflects the overall discriminatory ability of the marker, over time. In absence of censoring, the traditional KM estimator can be employed. If censoring is present, the estimates described in the previous subsection are recommended.

6.4.4 Incident/static

Under the following definition, a subject does not change disease status:

$$sensitivity^I(c,t) : P(X_i > c|\mathcal{T}_i = t) = TPR_t^I \tag{6.23}$$

$$specificity^D(c,t^*) : P(X_i \leq c|\mathcal{T}_i > t^*) = 1 - FPR_{t^*}^D. \tag{6.24}$$

Controls are those subjects that are event free at $(0, t^*)$ and cases are defined as such according to the time at which the event occurs. The derivation of the ROC curve is straightforward once we have both the sensitivity and specificity. The AUC can also be straightforwardly calculated at a time point t. This definition is presented by Etzioni et al. (1999) [80], and Slate and Turnbull (2000) [248], where parametric regression models that facilitate $\mathcal{T}_i = t$ as a covariate are studied. Cai et al. (2006) [46] present methods that further accommodate censoring while Zheng and Heagerty (2004) [306] consider models that relax parametric assumptions.

6.4.5 Incident/dynamic

Under this definition, we have

$$sensitivityI(c,t) : P(X_i > c|\mathcal{T}_i = t) = TPR_t^I \tag{6.25}$$

$$specificity^D(c,t) : P(X_i \leq c|\mathcal{T}_i > t^*) = 1 - FPR_t^D. \tag{6.26}$$

It is easy to see that under this definition an individual that is initially considered as a control at early times, it may be considered as a case when $t = \mathcal{T}_i$. As pointed out in Heagerty and Zheng (2005) [117], the sensitivity is the expected fraction of subjects with $X > c$ among the subpopulation of subjects that die at time t. The specificity in turn is the fraction of subjects with $X < c$ among those who live beyond t. One advantage of this definition compared to the previous ones is the relation to hazard rate modeling since the incident sensitivity and dynamic specificity are defined based on the risk set at time t. Another advantage is related to the accommodation of longitudinal biomarker measurements through a sensitivity defined by $P(X_i(t) > c|\mathcal{T}_i = t)$ and a specificity defined by $P(X_i(t) \leq c|\mathcal{T}_i > t)$.

6.5 Exercises

6.1 The package `ROCnReg` [223] in `R` implements a large number of existing approaches for ROC regression outlined in this chapter. Explore the function `cROC.sp` to assess the accuracy of `ALB` in discriminating between healthy subjects and pancreatitis patients adjusting for the effect of `A1GL`.

6.2 Using `ROCnReg`, explore the use of the function `pooledROC.emp` for the assessment of the accuracy of `ALB` in discriminating between healthy subjects and pancreatitis patients.

6.3 Interpret the output (parameter estimates) of the `R`-code provided in Section 6.2.4 relative to the corresponding ROC curve.

6.4 Using the Late-onset sepsis data, assess the effect of TREM1 on the diagnostic accuracy of IL6 in discriminating between sepsis and no-sepsis subjects. Then, assess the combined diagnostic accuracy of IL6 and TREM1 using logistic regression. Interpret the results.

7

Missing Data and Errors-in-Variables in ROC Analysis

CONTENTS

7.1 ROC Analysis under Verification Bias 161
7.1.1 Verification bias in binary test evaluation 162
7.1.1.1 Illustration using R 164
7.1.2 Verification bias in ROC curve estimation 168
7.1.3 Verification bias for three class (ROC surface) analysis 170
7.1.3.1 Implementation using R 171
7.2 Marker Measurements in the Presence of a Limit of Detection . 174
7.2.1 Empirical ROC for markers with LoD 174
7.2.2 Parametric models for markers with LoD: Box-Cox and the extended generalized gamma ROC curves 175
7.2.3 A hybrid approach 177
7.3 ROC Analysis with Measurement Error 177
7.3.1 Parametric analysis for markers with measurement error 178
7.4 ROC Analysis under Imperfect Reference Standard Bias 179
7.4.1 Binary markers under an imperfect reference standard . 180
7.4.2 Non-binary markers under an imperfect reference standard 182
7.5 Exercises 183

7.1 ROC Analysis under Verification Bias

In many settings, it is not feasible or even ethical to obtain the reference status information for all individuals in order to assess the diagnostic performance of the marker. For example, subjects/subgroups that are considered to have a higher risk of having the disease are more likely to undergo the process of the reference standard. Thus, using only those data points that correspond to individuals for which the reference standard results are available might result in biased estimates of diagnostic performance. This type of bias is known as *verification bias.* We stress here the dual potential downside from ignoring

DOI: 10.1201/9780429170140-7

missing data: on the one hand, there is the potential for bias and on the other, there is the subtler potential to underestimate the uncertainty of the estimates because of the missing information.

Accounting for verification bias when estimating accuracy measures such as sensitivity, specificity, NPV, and PPV requires assumptions about the missing data mechanism and, specifically here, the reference standard missingness mechanism. In the statistical literature, we distinguish three classes of missing data according to the mechanism that generates missingness. In particular, data are said to be *missing completely at random (MCAR)* if the missing data are unrelated to the available study variables. For example, the missing reference standard does not depend on any of the known characteristics of the cases. Data are said to be *missing at random (MAR)* when the missing data depend only on the available study variables. For example, the missing true disease status depends only on the observed data. Missing at random means there might be systematic differences between the missing and observed values, but these can be entirely explained by other observed variables, such as the marker measurements *per se*. A third catefory of missingness is *missing not at random (MNAR)*, which implies that the available variables do not account for differences in the distribution of the missing variables between observed and missing cases. For example, the missing true disease status may depend on characteristics of the case that are not captured in the study variables. These assumptions are discussed in detail in the classic book by Little and Rubin (2002) [152], which presents a variety of methods for handling missingness, including multiple imputation. A systematic review of the different approaches in the diagnostic testing setting is reported in Umemneku Chikere et al. (2019) [268].

7.1.1 Verification bias in binary test evaluation

To fix ideas, we use an illustrative example from the literature [6]. The general structure of the data is presented in Table 7.1. The table shows the observed data from a study of $n = n_2 + n_1$ subjects in which the reference standard is not obtained in u_2 cases with a positive test result and u_1 cases with a negative test result.

The setting is the assessment of test sensitivity and specificity in a study of $n = 1000$ participants from a population in which disease prevalence is $p = P(D = 2) = 0.10$. The actual values of sensitivity and specificity are 80% and 90%, respectively. If all test and reference status data were available, the resulting table is given on the left-hand side of Table 7.2. If the reference standard is obtained only for 10% of the cases with a negative test result but for all cases with a positive test result, the table would be as shown on the right-hand side of Table 7.2. Designs for which all cases testing positive undergo verification but only a subset of those testing negative do so are commonly used.

TABLE 7.1
Data structure for the verification bias problem when T is dichotomous. V is a binary indicator of the availability of the reference standard, with $V = 1$ when the reference standard is available and $V = 0$ otherwise.

V	D	$T = 2$	$T = 1$
1	2	s_2	s_1
1	1	r_2	r_1
0	Missing	u_2	u_1
	Total:	n_2	n_1

TABLE 7.2
Example presented in Alonzo and Pepe (2005) [6]. Left side: results when disease verification is obtained for everyone. Right side: observed data when disease verification is obtained for all subjects who test positive and only 10% of subjects who test negative. V is a binary indicator of the availability of the reference standard.

V	D	$T = 2$	$T = 1$
1	2	80	20
1	1	90	810
0	Missing	0	0
	Total:	170	830

V	D	$T = 2$	$T = 1$
1	2	80	2
1	1	90	81
0	Missing	0	747
	Total:	170	830

A "complete case" analysis of the data, that is an analysis based only on the cases with both test and reference standard information, would result in an estimated (observed) sensitivity of $s_2/(s_2 + s_1) = 80/82$ or 98% and an estimated (observed) specificity of $r_1/(r_1 + r_2) = 81/171$ or 47%. This illustrates that if test positives are more likely to receive disease verification than test negatives, observed sensitivity overestimates true sensitivity (98% vs. 80%) and observed specificity underestimates true specificity (47% vs. 90%).

A simple calculation shows that, using the complete case data, the PPV, that is, $P(D = 2|T = 2)$ would be estimated as 47% and the NPV, that is $P(D = 1|T = 1)$ would be estimated as 98%. The reader would note here that these estimates are identical to those that would be obtained if there were no missing data in the reference information. The reason for this phenomenon is that PPV and NPV are defined conditionally on the test result and that the counts in the cells for $T = 1, V = 1$ of the second table are equal to the counts in the first table divided by 10. In other words, the proportion of verified cases for $T = 1$ is assumed the same across diseased and non-diseased cases. A detailed discussion of the effect of verification bias on estimates of positive and negative predictive values is presented in Zhou (1994) [309].

We now consider the question of correcting the bias in the estimates of sensitivity and specificity. A simple approach was introduced by Begg and Greenes (1983) [29] and employs Bayes' rule. For sensitivity, we obtain:

$$
\begin{aligned}
P(T=2|D=2) &= \frac{P(D=2|T=2)P(T=2)}{P(D=2|T=2)P(T=2)+P(D=2|T=1)P(T=1)} \\
&= \frac{\frac{s_2 n_2}{s_2+r_2}}{\frac{s_2 n_2}{s_2+r_2}+\frac{s_1 n_1}{s_1+r_1}}.
\end{aligned}
$$

Likewise, for specificity, we obtain:

$$
P(T=1|D=1) = \frac{\frac{r_1 n_1}{s_1+r_1}}{\frac{r_1 n_1}{s_1+r_1}+\frac{r_2 n_2}{s_2+r_2}}
$$

In effect, the above approach is a *single imputation* method. Multiple imputation approaches assume MAR missingness for the reference standard information. As discussed in Harel and Zhou (2006, 2007) [107,108], each missing data point is replaced by M imputed data points. Then these M imputed datasets are analyzed as if they are fully observed data. The multiple imputation method seems to be preferable when the missingness mechanism cannot be determined.

If the MAR assumption is not justifiable, alternative approaches have been discussed in the literature. In particular, Zhou (1993) [308] extended the work of Begg and Greenes (1983) [29] to accommodate less strict assumptions regarding the missingness mechanism. Another approach is given by Kosinski and Barhhart (2003) [141] that is based on deriving the region of sensitivity and specificity pairs that define the so-called ignorance region. An online tool is available for this approach at `http://uwmsk.org/gsa`.

7.1.1.1 Illustration using `R`

Using the `PVBcorrect` package [7] which can be downloaded from the website `https://github.com/wnarifin/PVBcorrect`, we illustrate methods of this section with a dataset involving patients with coronary artery disease (CAD). The single-photon-emission computed-tomography (SPECT) thallium test is a non-invasive test that can be used to diagnose CAD. CAD is diagnosed if coronary angiography indicates a stenosis of $> 50\%$ in an artery. This is an invasive reference standard. The discussed dataset is also described and elaborated in detail in Arifin and Yusof (2022) [7].

The dataset involves the following variables: 1. T (a binary SPECT test result, here 1=Positive, 0=Negative), 2. D (the binary reference standard for CAD, here 1=Yes, 0=No), and the following covariates: i. Gender (X_1 : 1=Male, 0=Female), ii. Stress mode (X_2 : 1=Dipyridamole, 0=Exercise), iii.

Age (X_3: Age, 1=60 years and above, 0=below 60). Dipyradomole is an antiplatelet medicine which prevents a type of blood cell (platelets) sticking together and forming blood clots.

In this dataset, 2688 patients underwent the SPECT thallium test but the CAD status was only verified on 471 patients (2217 or 82.5% of patients were unverified; thus the variable D (disease status) contains 2217 missing observations. The dataset is named `cad_pvb`.

```
summary(cad_pvb)
```

```
##          X1             X2              X3
## Min.     :0.0000   Min.    :0.000  Min.    :0.0000
## 1st Qu.  :0.0000   1st Qu. :0.000  1st Qu. :0.0000
## Median   :1.0000   Median  :0.000  Median  :0.0000
## Mean     :0.5737   Mean    :0.394  Mean    :0.4226
## 3rd Qu.  :1.0000   3rd Qu. :1.000  3rd Qu. :1.0000
## Max.     :1.0000   Max.    :1.000  Max.    :1.0000
##
##           T               D
## Min.     :0.0000       :0.0000
## 1st Qu.  :0.0000       :0.0000
## Median   :1.0000       :0.0000
## Mean     :0.5294       :0.4246
## 3rd Qu.  :1.0000       :1.0000
## Max.     :1.0000       :1.0000
## NA's                   :2217
```

The simplest approach, which can be used in the complete case analysis, is based only on the verified cases. Such an approach is unbiased under the MCAR mechanism [49,270] and is biased in the presence of partial verification bias [7]. Using the conventional notation in this book, the relevant sensitivity, specificity, PPV, and NPV estimates under the complete case approach (CCA) are given below:

$$\begin{aligned}
\hat{Se}_{CCA} = \hat{P}(T=2|D=2) &= \frac{s_2}{s_2+s_1} \\
\hat{Se}_{CCA} = \hat{P}(T=1|D=1) &= \frac{r_1}{r_2+r_1} \\
P\hat{P}V_{CCA} = \hat{P}(D=2|T=2) &= \frac{s_2}{s_2+r_2} \\
N\hat{P}V_{CCA} = \hat{P}(D=1|T=1) &= \frac{r_1}{s_1+r_1}.
\end{aligned}$$

The corresponding $100(1-\alpha)\%$ Wald confidence intervals are

$$\hat{Se}_{CCA} \pm z_{1-\alpha/2}\sqrt{\frac{s_2 s_1}{(s_2+s_1)^3}}$$
$$\hat{Sp}_{CCA} \pm z_{1-\alpha/2}\sqrt{\frac{r_2 r_1}{(r_2+r_1)^3}}$$
$$\widehat{PPV}_{CCA} \pm z_{1-\alpha/2}\sqrt{\frac{s_2 r_2}{(s_2+r_2)^3}}$$
$$\widehat{NPV}_{CCA} \pm z_{1-\alpha/2}\sqrt{\frac{s_1 r_1}{(s_1+r_1)^3}}.$$

The cross-classification table can be obtained by the function `view_table` of the `PVBcorrect` package:

```
view_table(data = cad_pvb, test = "T", disease = "D")
```

```
##       Disease
## Test   yes   no
## yes    195  232
## no       5   39
```

The `acc_cca` function can provide the aforementioned estimates along with their 95% CIs:

```
cca_out = acc_cca(data = cad_pvb, test = "T", disease = "D", ci = T)
cca_est = cca_out$acc_results
cca_est
```

```
## Estimates of accuracy measures
## Uncorrected for PVB: Complete Case Analysis
##              Est         SE     LowCI     UppCI
## Sn     0.9750000 0.01103970 0.9533626 0.9966374
## Sp     0.1439114 0.02132173 0.1021216 0.1857013
## PPV    0.4566745 0.02410569 0.4094282 0.5039207
## NPV    0.8863636 0.04784519 0.7925888 0.9801385
```

An extension of the Begg and Greenes method (BG) discussed above refers to the Extended Begg and Greens (EBG) method [6]. The EBG method is applicable under the MAR assumption and implies the following estimates in the presence of a covariate Z_i:

$$\widehat{Se}_{EBG} = \frac{\sum_{i=1}^{n} T_i \hat{P}(D_i = 2|T_i, Z_i)}{\sum_{i=1}^{n} \hat{P}(D_i = 2|T_i, Z_i)} \quad (7.1)$$

$$\widehat{Sp}_{EBG} = \frac{\sum_{i=1}^{n} (1 - T_i)[1 - \hat{P}(D_i = 2|T_i, Z_i)}{\sum_{i=1}^{n} 1 - \hat{P}(D_i = 2|T_i, Z_i)} \quad (7.2)$$

where $\hat{P}(D_i = 2|T_i, Z_i)$ can be derived through a logistic regression model. Using Bayes' theorem, we also get:

$$\widehat{PPV}_{EBG} = \frac{\hat{P}(D = 2) \times \hat{Se}_{EBG}}{\hat{P}(D = 2) \times \hat{Se}_{EBG} + \hat{P}(D = 1) \times (1 - \hat{Sp}_{EBG})} \quad (7.3)$$

$$\widehat{NPV}_{EBG} = \frac{\hat{P}(D = 1) \times \hat{Sp}_{EBG}}{\hat{P}(D = 1) \times \hat{Sp}_{EBG} + \hat{P}(D = 2) \times (1 - \hat{Se}_{EBG})}. \quad (7.4)$$

A bootstrap approach for the derivation of the corresponding standard errors and CIs is described in Arifin and Yusof (2022) [7].

Through the function acc_ebg, we can obtain the EBG estimates along with their 95% CIs.

```
ebg_out = acc_ebg(data = cad_pvb, test = "T", disease = "D",
ci = TRUE, ci_type = "bca", seednum = 12345, R = 999)
ebg_est = ebg_out$acc_results
ebg_est
```

```
## Estimates of accuracy measures
## Corrected for PVB: Extended Begg and Greenes' Method
##           Est         SE    LowCI     UppCI
## Sn  0.8188629 0.06438696 0.6808328 0.9305696
## Sp  0.5918754 0.01759285 0.5538231 0.6241082
## PPV 0.4566745 0.02421467 0.4090813 0.5083287
## NPV 0.8863636 0.04925696 0.7662900 0.9605648
```

Using the EBG method with covariate X_3 implies:

```
ebgx_out = acc_ebg(data = cad_pvb, test = "T", disease = "D",
covariate = "X3", saturated_model = TRUE, ci = TRUE,
ci_type = "bca", seednum = 12345, R = 999)
ebgx_est = ebgx_out$acc_results
ebgx_est
```

```
##            Est          SE     LowCI     UppCI
## Sn  0.8400495 0.06060738 0.6968409 0.9360124
## Sp  0.5912022 0.01573772 0.5566062 0.6194934
## PPV 0.4437285 0.02342825 0.3993989 0.4935086
## NPV 0.9049587 0.04311795 0.7883877 0.9669421
```

The option `saturated_model`, when set as TRUE, allows the user to get results that are equivalent to the BG method through the use of a saturated model.

Harel and Zhou (2006) [107] discuss a multiple imputation-based method as an alternative. It involves repeated imputation of missing values through the posterior predictive distribution. This method is also included in the software provided by Arifin and Yosuf (2022) [7]. Another alternative that incorporates data under a MNAR mechanism that is also provided by the same software is discussed in Kosinski and Barnhart (2003) [140]. They propose a method using logistic regression models under an EM algorithm to correct for partial verification bias under a MNAR mechanism. For further details about the implementation of these in `R`, we refer the interested reader to the work of Arifin and Yosuf (2022) [7].

7.1.2 Verification bias in ROC curve estimation

Selective availability of the reference standard information can also create bias in ROC estimation. An ROC curve estimate yields an unbiased estimate if the reference standard is MCAR. When the missingness mechanism is MAR, then bias correction approaches must be employed. Such approaches are discussed in Alonzo and Pepe (2005) [6] and are based on different imputation techniques as well as the so-called inverse probability weighting (IPW) approach. We briefly refer to both.

The first imputation approach is called the full imputation (FI) method. This involves imputing $\rho = P(D|X, Z)$ for all individuals which implies that the estimated sensitivity and specificity are given by:

$$\widehat{TPR}_{FI}(c) = \frac{\sum_{i=1}^{n} I(X_i \geq c)\hat{\rho}_i}{\sum_{i=1}^{n} \hat{\rho}_i}, \qquad \widehat{FPR}_{FI}(c) = \frac{\sum_{i=1}^{n} I(X_i \geq c)(1-\hat{\rho}_i)}{\sum_{i=1}^{n}(1-\hat{\rho}_i)},$$

where $\hat{\rho}_i = \hat{P}(D_i = 1|X_i, Z_i)$ which can be obtained through logistic regression. Plotting the FPR and TPR in the unit square will result in the visualization of the corresponding ROC estimate and the underlying AUC estimate can be obtained using the trapezoidal rule of integration as in Bamber (1975) [10]. This strategy can also be applied for the remaining imputation approaches for the derivation of the underlying AUC estimate.

Another approach involves mean score imputation (MSI) that involves imputing the disease status for those individuals that the reference standard is not available, while we use the available disease status for those individuals that the reference standard is available. The corresponding TPR and FPR are given by:

$$\widehat{TPR}_{MSI}(c) = \frac{\sum_{i=1}^{n} I(X_i \geq c)\{V_i D_i + (1 - V_i)\hat{\rho}_i\}}{\sum_{i=1}^{n}\{V_i D_i + (1 - V_i)\hat{\rho}_i\}}$$

$$\widehat{FPR}_{MSI}(c) = \frac{\sum_{i=1}^{n} I(X_i \geq c)\{V_i(1 - D_i) + (1 - V_i)(1 - \hat{\rho}_i)\}}{\sum_{i=1}^{n}\{V_i(1 - D_i) + (1 - V_i)(1 - \hat{\rho}_i)\}}.$$

An alternative approach, known as the IPW approach, was first introduced under a regression framework by Horvitz and Thompson (1952) [125] and is discussed under a verification bias setting by Alonzo and Pepe (2005) [6]. Under this setting, the weights are the inverse of the probability of an individual being selected for verification with the reference standard. Intuitively, if this probability is very small, then the weight is going to exhibit a large value so that it allows for adequate representation of such individuals in the sample. For such a strategy, the TPR and FPR are given by:

$$\widehat{TPR}_{IPW}(c) = \frac{\sum_{i=1}^{n} I(X_i \geq c) V_i D_i / \hat{\pi}_i}{\sum_{i=1}^{n} V_i D_i / \hat{\pi}_i}$$

$$\widehat{FPR}_{IPW}(c) = \frac{\sum_{i=1}^{n} I(X_i \geq c) V_i(1 - D_i)/\hat{\pi}_i}{\sum_{i=1}^{n} V_i(1 - D_i)/\hat{\pi}_i},$$

where $\hat{\pi} = P(V_i|X_i, Z_i)$. In He et al. (2009) [110], a closed form expression for the underlying AUC is provided. Finally, the doubly robust (DR) estimators are also presented in Alonzo and Pepe (2005) [6]:

$$\widehat{TPR}_{DR}(c) = \frac{\sum_{i=1}^{n} I(X_i \geq c)\{V_i D_i/\hat{\pi}_i - (V_i - \hat{\pi}_i)\hat{\rho}_i/\hat{\pi}_i\}}{\sum_{i=1}^{n}\{V_i D_i/\hat{\pi}_i - (V_i - \hat{\pi}_i)\hat{\rho}_i/\hat{\pi}_i\}},$$

$$\widehat{FPR}_{DR}(c) = \frac{\sum_{i=1}^{n} I(X_i \geq c)\{V_i(1 - D_i)/\hat{\pi}_i - (V_i - \hat{\pi}_i)(1 - \hat{\rho}_i)/\hat{\pi}_i\}}{\sum_{i=1}^{n}\{V_i(1 - D_i)/\hat{\pi}_i - (V_i - \hat{\pi}_i)(1 - \hat{\rho}_i)/\hat{\pi}_i\}}.$$

The advantage of the latter approach is that the TPR and FPR estimates are consistent if consistent estimators are available for either π_i or ρ_i. This implies that the verification model can be miss-specified yet the TPR and FPR estimates, and as a result the ROC estimate, will still be consistent. For this reason, Alonzo and Pepe (2005) [6] recommend these estimators over the ones previously discussed.

Further approaches which address the issue of verification bias involve bayesian techniques [162], accommodation of covariates that are also affected by the verification bias [222], comparison of continuous tests [310], and binary tests [227] in the presence of verification bias, as well as issues that relate to the estimation of the NPV and the PPV [309].

7.1.3 Verification bias for three class (ROC surface) analysis

Extending the implications of verification bias to a three-class setting involves the task of obtaining unbiased estimators of the underlying ROC surface and the implied VUS [261]. We assume that the verification status V and the disease status D are mutually independent given the test result X (and potential covariates Z). That is, $P(V|X, Z) = P(V|D, X, Z)$ or equivalently $P(D|X, Z) = P(D|X, V, Z)$ which is a special case of the MAR assumption [152].

Under the MAR assumption, as discussed in To et al. (2016) [260], we have

$$
\begin{aligned}
T\hat{C}F_{1,FI} &= 1 - \frac{\sum_{i=1}^{n} I(X_i > c_1)\hat{\rho}_{1i}}{\sum_{i=1}^{n} \hat{\rho}_{1i}}, \\
T\hat{C}F_{2,FI} &= \frac{\sum_{i=1}^{n} I(c_1 < X_i < c_2)\hat{\rho}_{2i}}{\sum_{i=1}^{n} \hat{\rho}_{2i}}, \\
T\hat{C}F_{3,FI} &= \frac{\sum_{i=1}^{n} I(X_i > c_2)\hat{\rho}_{3i}}{\sum_{i=1}^{n} \hat{\rho}_{3i}},
\end{aligned}
$$

where $\rho_{ki} = P(D_{ki} = 1|X_i, Z_i)$ and its estimate $\hat{\rho}_{ki}$ can be obtained using only data from verified individuals. This can be done through an assumed model such as the multinomial logistic regression model. An alternative MSI approach employs the estimated $\hat{\rho}_{ki}$ only for the missing values of the disease status D_{ki} and yields:

$$
\begin{aligned}
T\hat{C}F_{1,MSI} &= 1 - \frac{\sum_{i=1}^{n} I(X_i > c_1)[V_i I(D_{1i} = 1) + (1 - V_i)\hat{\rho}_{1i}]}{\sum_{i=1}^{n}[V_i I(D_{1i} = 1) + (1 - V_i)\hat{\rho}_{1i}]}, \\
T\hat{C}F_{2,MSI} &= \frac{\sum_{i=1}^{n} I(c_1 < X_i < c_2)[V_i I(D_{2i} = 1) + (1 - V_i)\hat{\rho}_{2i}]}{\sum_{i=1}^{n}[V_i I(D_{2i} = 1) + (1 - V_i)\hat{\rho}_{2i}]}, \\
T\hat{C}F_{3,MSI} &= \frac{\sum_{i=1}^{n} I(X_i > c_2)[V_i I(D_{3i} = 1) + (1 - V_i)\hat{\rho}_{3i}]}{\sum_{i=1}^{n}[V_i I(D_{3i} = 1) + (1 - V_i)\hat{\rho}_{3i}]}.
\end{aligned}
$$

Another approach, which weighs each individual for which $V_i = 1$ by the inverse probability that the subject is selected, is referred to as IPW and the corresponding TCF estimates are given by:

$$
\begin{aligned}
T\hat{C}F_{1,IPW} &= 1 - \frac{\sum_{i=1}^{n} I(X_i > c_1)V_i\hat{\pi}_i^{-1}I(D_{1i} = 1)}{\sum_{i=1}^{n} V_i\hat{\pi}_i^{-1}I(D_{1i} = 1)}, \\
T\hat{C}F_{2,IPW} &= \frac{\sum_{i=1}^{n} I(c_1 < X_i < c_2)V_i\hat{\pi}_i^{-1}I(D_{2i} = 2)}{\sum_{i=1}^{n} V_i\hat{\pi}_i^{-1}I(D_{2i} = 2)}, \\
T\hat{C}F_{3,IPW} &= \frac{\sum_{i=1}^{n} I(X_i > c_2)V_i\hat{\pi}_i^{-1}I(D_{3i} = 3)}{\sum_{i=1}^{n} V_i\hat{\pi}_i^{-1}I(D_{3i} = 3)}.
\end{aligned}
$$

The IPW version of the TCFs weighs each individual by the inverse probability of being selected. This implies the following estimates:

$$
\begin{aligned}
\hat{TCF}_{1,SPE} &= 1 - \frac{\sum_{i=1}^{n} I(X_i > c_1)\left(\frac{V_i I(D_{1i}=1)}{\hat{\pi}_i} - \frac{\hat{\rho}_{1i} V_i - \hat{\pi}_i}{\hat{\pi}_i}\right)}{\sum_{i=1}^{n}\left(\frac{V_i I(D_{1i}=1)}{\hat{\pi}_i} - \frac{\hat{\rho}_{1i} V_i - \hat{\pi}_i}{\hat{\pi}_i}\right)} \\
\hat{TCF}_{1,SPE} &= \frac{\sum_{i=1}^{n} I(c_1 < X_i < c_2)\left(\frac{V_i I(D_{2i}=2)}{\hat{\pi}_i} - \frac{\hat{\rho}_{2i} V_i - \hat{\pi}_i}{\hat{\pi}_i}\right)}{\sum_{i=1}^{n}\left(\frac{V_i I(D_{2i}=2)}{\hat{\pi}_i} - \frac{\hat{\rho}_{2i} V_i - \hat{\pi}_i}{\hat{\pi}_i}\right)} \\
\hat{TCF}_{3,SPE} &= \frac{\sum_{i=1}^{n} I(X_i > c_2)\left(\frac{V_i I(D_{3i}=3)}{\hat{\pi}_i} - \frac{\hat{\rho}_{3i} V_i - \hat{\pi}_i}{\hat{\pi}_i}\right)}{\sum_{i=1}^{n}\left(\frac{V_i I(D_{3i}=3)}{\hat{\pi}_i} - \frac{\hat{\rho}_{3i} V_i - \hat{\pi}_i}{\hat{\pi}_i}\right)},
\end{aligned}
$$

where $\hat{\pi}_i$ is an estimate of the conditional verification probabilities, i.e. $\hat{\pi}_i = P(V_i = 1|X_i, Z_i)$.

The MSI, IPW, and SPE estimators are extensions of the two class case estimators presented in Alonzo and Pepe (2005) [6]. Notice that the SPE estimators can lie outside the $(0, 1)$ interval since $\left(\frac{V_i I(D_{3i}=3)}{\hat{\pi}_i} - \frac{\hat{\rho}_{3i} V_i - \hat{\pi}_i}{\hat{\pi}_i}\right)$ can take negative values as well. A nearest neighbor nonparametric estimator has also been proposed in To et al. (2020) [261].

7.1.3.1 Implementation using R

In this section, we briefly discuss the `bcROCsurface` package [258]. Its usage allows us to employ all five methods discussed above, i.e. the full imputation (FI), the MSI, the IPW, the semiparametric efficient (SPE), and the K-nearest neighbor (KNN). The bias correction techniques apply on the ROC surface and its VUS and the package refers to continuous biomarkers. Note that utilization of these methods is valid if the missingness mechanism is MAR. The data need to include i) the variable that represents the disease status (with three classes), ii) the biomarker values, iii) the binary variable of the verification status (1 for verified 0 for not verified), and iv) other covariates. Some packages need to be pre-loaded, then a basic description of the dataset used for this illustration is given. We use the dataset illustrated in To (2017) [258] and discussed in detail in To et al. (2016) [260]. It involves patients with ovarian cancer. Two biomarkers are available, CA125 and CA153 along with age as a covariate.

```
library("stats")
library("nnet")
library("rgl")
library("boot")
```

```
library("utils")
library("graphics")
library("parallel")
library("bcROCsurface")

# Loading the attached dataset
data(EOC)
head(EOC)
```

```
##   D.full V  D        CA125       CA153 Age
## 1      3 1  3  3.304971965  1.42822875  41
## 2      1 0 NA  0.112479444  0.11665310  52
## 3      2 1  2  2.375011262 -0.04096794  50
## 4      1 0 NA -0.001545381  0.32111633  66
## 5      1 0 NA  0.278200345 -0.14283052  52
## 6      2 0 NA  0.167645382  0.81470563  50
```

Note that in the above dataset, the column that refers to the disease status exhibits multiple "NA" values, as expected. These refer to the unverified individuals which the correspond to a V value of zero. Usage of this package involves some data preparation that involves using the function `preDATA()`. This function allows the user to be informed as to whether the package can be employed on the available data. The control process involves the ordering of the three underlying groups as well as the existence of "NA" values on the disease status variables.

In the above example, the package is employed to evaluate the accuracy of ovarian cancer-related tumor marker CA125. Here CA125 will be the diagnostic test of interest, CA153 and Age will be the two auxiliary covariates. V is the verification status, and D is the disease status.

First the prerequisites for the appropriate use of the package are verified.

```
dise<-preDATA(EOC$D, EOC$CA125)
```

The verification probabilities below can be obtained through the function `psglm()` which employs a generalized linear model. The choices are logistic, probit, or a threshold regression model, with the logistic model being the default. The disease probabilities can be obtained through the functions `rhoMLogit()` and `rhoKNN()` which utilize a multinomial logistic regression model.

```
#Defining the missing disease status
EOC$dise.gpr<-dise$D
EOC$dise.mat<-dise$Dvec

# Estimate the disease probabilities
rho.out <- rhoMLogit(dise.gpr ~ CA125 + CA153 + Age,data = EOC)
#rho.out

# Estimate the verification probabilites
pi.out <- psglm(V ~ CA125 + CA153 + Age,data = EOC)
#pi.out
```

For inference involving the VUS, the function `vus()` can be used.

```
vus.fi <- vus(method = "fi", T = EOC$CA125,
              Dvec = EOC$dise.mat, V = EOC$V,
              rhoEst = rho.out, ci = TRUE)
vus.fi
```

```
## CALL: vus(method = "fi", T = EOC$CA125, Dvec = EOC$dise.mat, V = EOC$V,
##     rhoEst = rho.out, ci = TRUE)

## Estimate of VUS: 0.515
## Standard error: 0.0404

## Intervals:
## Level         Normal                Logit
## 95%    ( 0.4357,  0.5942 )    ( 0.4360,  0.5932 )
## Estimation of Standard Error and Intervals are based on Asymptotic Theory

## Testing the null hypothesis H0: VUS = 1/6
##               Test Statistic   P-value
## Normal-test          8.6168 < 2.2e-16 ***
## ---
## Signif. codes:  0 '***' 0.001 '**' 0.01 '*' 0.05 '.' 0.1 ' ' 1
```

Estimates and confidence intervals for the VUS can be obtained by using the rest of the methods in a similar way.

7.2 Marker Measurements in the Presence of a Limit of Detection

In some cases, technological restrictions do not allow us to obtain biomarker measurements below an analytical concentration/quantification limit, known as the Limit of Detection (LoD). Usually, these settings involve a lower LoD implying the existence of left censoring. Denote the LoD by d_L and set measurements equal to d_L when the actual biomarker value is lower than this. In the case of an upper LoD, where measurements above a specific value cannot be quantified, denote the LoD by d_U. As a consequence, right-censored data arise.

When measurements subject to an LoD exist, in order to construct the corresponding ROC curve one needs to account for the censored nature of the data. In the presence of a lower LoD, common practice, outside the ROC analysis framework, suggests imputing measurements equal to d_L. In the simplest approach, these can be replaced with $d_L/2$ or with $d_L/\sqrt{2}$ (see e.g. [124,191]). However, these commonly used approaches ignore the occurrence of censoring, while in the ROC analysis framework, they actually result in the same empirical ROC curve estimates as with an approach that simply uses d_L. All these approaches are expected to result in biased estimates of the ROC curve and its respective indices.

A framework that may be useful and generally simple in such settings is to employ parametric models that account for the censored scores. The corresponding binormal and bigamma models have been discussed in the literature [88,182,207]. Maximum likelihood ratio tests are discussed in Vexler et al. (2008) [275], and the multivariate normality assumption is described in Perkins et al. (2013) [210] for settings where multiple biomarkers are subject to an LoD. Linear combinations of markers under an LoD setting are discussed in Perkins et al. (2011) [209]. In Bantis et al. (2012) [21], the three-class setting is addressed and methods for estimating an ROC surface are described. In the following sections, we will discuss the simple scenario where a single marker in subject to an LoD and interest lies in obtaining an estimate of the corresponding ROC curve.

7.2.1 Empirical ROC for markers with LoD

In the presence of an LoD, a direct approach is to construct the empirical ROC estimate and ignore the fact that some data are actually censored. Namely, deal with all data as if they were fully observed. As mentioned above, this is equivalent to imputing the data with any fixed replacement value that is lower than d_L when there is a lower limit of quantification and higher than d_U when there is an upper limit of quantification. More specifically, for any replacement value $\alpha_L < d_L$ and/or $\alpha_U > d_U$, the empirical estimate of the

ROC curve remains the same when it is obtained by an analysis that ignores the censored nature of the data.

In Perkins et al. (2007) [207], it is shown that in such cases the theoretical ROC is generally biased, while in Bantis et al. (2017) [24] this result is generalized in a framework that accommodates a lower LoD, an upper LoD, or both. In addition, they discuss which conditions imply the existence of a downward bias. However, it may be the case that, under some specific conditions, the imputation-based ROC, using a fixed replacement value for the censored scores, is unbiased. These conditions relate to the concavity of the true and generally unknown ROC curve [24].

Denote with ROC_M the ROC resulting from the censored scores M_1 and M_2 which in turn are based on simple (single) replacement values of a_L (and/or α_U in the case of an upper LoD). It is easy to show that ROC_M remains the same for any replacement value α_L and α_U. We further define ROC_M^* by linearly completing $ROC_M(t)$, illustrated as the "naive empirical" estimate in Figure 7.1. Then, for the corresponding AUC, denoted by AUC_M^* we have [24]:

$$AUC_M^* = \frac{S_1(d_U)S_2(d_U)}{2} + \int_{S_1(d_U)}^{S_1(d_L)} ROC(t)dt + \frac{(1 - S_1(d_L))(1 - S_2(d_L))}{2},$$

where $S_1 = 1 - F_1$ and $S_2 = 1 - F_2$ correspond to the non-diseased and diseased groups, respectively. AUC_M^* will be smaller than the AUC that would be obtained if the LoD measurements were observed, when the marker is subject to an upper LoD and $PPV(c)$ is increasing in c, or when the marker is subject to a lower LoD and $NPV(c)$ is decreasing in c, or when the marker is subject to both upper and lower LoDs and with $PPV(c)$ increasing and $NPV(c)$ decreasing in c.

Strictly speaking, the replacement value practice is valid when we are willing to make the assumption that, in terms of patient classification, knowledge of the actual marker measurement is useless when the process of classification involves classifying a patient as healthy based on a value smaller than the lower LoD or when classifying a patient as having the disease based on a value larger than the upper LoD. These are reasonable assumptions quite often in practice unless there is a high proportion of measurements subject to LoD [24].

7.2.2 Parametric models for markers with LoD: Box-Cox and the extended generalized gamma ROC curves

Using parametric models for the underlying distributions of diseased and non-diseased subjects offers an efficient framework for the accommodation of the censored nature of the data in the LoD context. Use of the binormal and the gamma model is discussed in Franco-Pereira et al. (2019) [88], while use of the extended generalized gamma (EGG) model along with the Box-Cox and

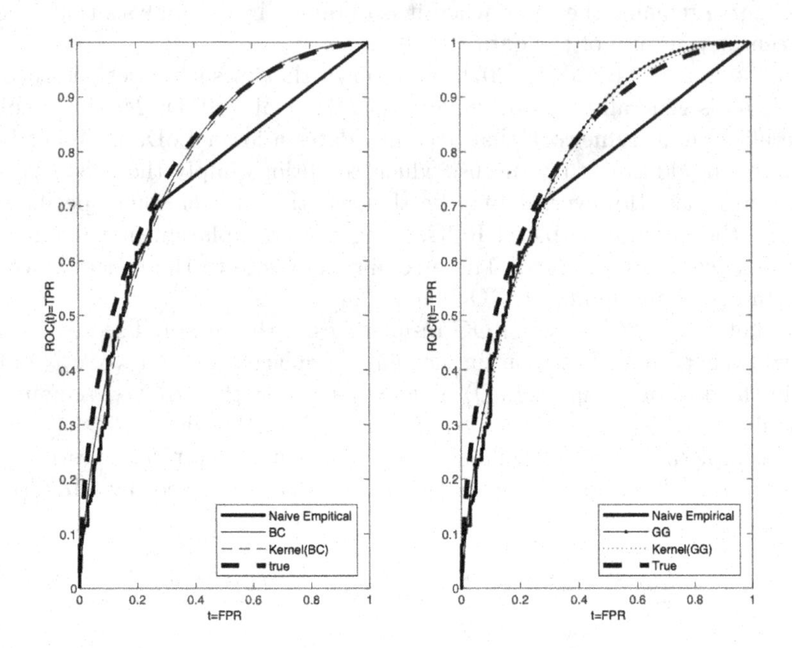

FIGURE 7.1
Simulated dataset of two normal distributions generated to attain true AUC=0.8 and expected level of censoring 50% due to a lower LoD. Left panel: Box-Cox (BC) and kernel(BC) hybrid *ROCs* along with the true ROC curve and the naive empirical estimate. Right panel: Generalized gamma (GG) and kernel(GG) hybrid along with the true ROC and the naive empirical.

hybrid parametric and kernel based methods are presented in Bantis et al. (2017) [24]. The EGG model density is,

$$f(x;\alpha,\lambda,\gamma)=\frac{|\alpha|}{\Gamma(\gamma)}\gamma^{\gamma}\lambda^{\alpha\gamma}x^{\alpha\gamma-1}exp\left\{-\gamma(\lambda x)^{\alpha}\right\},$$

where $\alpha \neq 0$ and $\gamma > 0$ are the shape parameters, and $\lambda > 0$ is the scale parameter. When $\alpha = 0$, the limiting case of the lognormal distribution is obtained. When $\gamma = 1$ or $\alpha = 1$, we obtain the Weibull or the gamma distribution, respectively. The respective survival function is

$$S(x;\alpha,\lambda,\gamma)=\begin{cases} I\left\{\gamma(\lambda x)^{\alpha},\gamma\right\}, & \text{if } \alpha<0 \\ 1-I\left\{\gamma(\lambda x)^{\alpha},\gamma\right\}, & \text{if } \alpha>0. \end{cases}$$

where $I\{\cdot,\cdot\}$ is the incomplete gamma function, defined as $I(x,\theta) = \frac{1}{\Gamma(\theta)}\int_0^x t^{\theta-1}e^{-t}dt$. The hazard rate of this density is flexible enough to accommodate the four most common types of hazard, i.e., increasing, decreasing, arc-shaped, and bathtub-shaped. The Extended Generalized Gamma (EGG-based) ROC curve can be derived after considering the maximum likelihood estimates of the involved parameters. For the technical details and a discussion about the EGG-based ROC, we refer the reader to Bantis et al. (2017) [24]. Relevant code for this implementation can be found in `www.leobantis.net`.

7.2.3 A hybrid approach

A hybrid approach discussed in Bantis et al. (2017) [24] is based on using both a nonparametric kernel estimate and a parametric model. Emphasis is given on the parametric model for completing the tail through multiple imputation [152], while the main body of the ROC curve is based on a nonparametric kernel-based estimator that is constructed from the fully observed part of the data. This hybrid approach involves imputing the censored data by random draws of plausible parametric models in order to obtain *pseudo-data* in the tails of both distributions, namely, for both the diseased and the non-diseased group. Then, one proceeds with the nonparametric kernel-based estimators for both distributions separately and hence obtain an estimate of the resulting kernel-based ROC.

A plot of some plausible parametric models that can be used alone or in combination with the kernel estimate is illustrated in Figure 7.1.

7.3 ROC Analysis with Measurement Error

Up to this point, we have been relying on the assumption that the biomarker scores, even for poorly performing markers, were accurately measured. However, there are settings in practice where measurement error is present. This implies that the measurements themselves are not an accurate representation of the true measurements of an individual. This error/variability could be due to laboratory conditions, technology limitations, as well as training of the operators of the involved instruments. Examples in which measurement errors may be induced by the laboratory instruments or even their operators have been presented in the literature [48, 53], such as measuring blood pressure in children where the measurement heavily depends on the operator. This is a different setting than the LoD one of Section 7.2, where LoD measurements are due to instrument/technological limitations.

Random measurement error can bias our estimators of the AUC and the ROC-related measures in general. Faraggi (2000) [82] discusses the effect of random measurement error on the confidence interval for the AUC in the binormal setting. He shows that not taking measurement error into account may yield seriously misleading results that, in turn, may imply a severe underestimation of the performance of the studied marker. Such underestimation will typically result in poor coverage properties of the confidence intervals around the AUC.

In this section, we present an approach to estimation of the AUC and the underlying corrected confidence intervals under the binormal model where random measurement error is accounted for [234]. When the normality assumption cannot be justified by the data at hand, a nonparametric alternative was proposed by Coffin and Sukhatme (1997) [53]. The latter approach can also be considered as a nonparametric alternative for bias correction when interest lies in AUC estimation.

7.3.1 Parametric analysis for markers with measurement error

Recall that, under the binormal model, assuming that $X_1 \sim N(\mu_1, \sigma_2^2)$ and $X_2 \sim N(\mu_2, \sigma_2^2)$, the AUC can be written as:

$$AUC = \Phi\left(\frac{\mu_2 - \mu_1}{\sqrt{\sigma_1^2 + \sigma_2^2}}\right)$$

In the presence of measurement error, the true biomarker value is not available. Instead, we have a score that is contaminated by measurement error and, thus, under the extra assumption that this error is random, we consider that the data are generated by the following mechanism:

$$\begin{aligned} x_{1i} &= X_{1i} + \epsilon_{1i}, \quad i = 1, 2, \ldots, n_1 \\ x_{2i} &= X_{2i} + \epsilon_{2i}, \quad i = 1, 2, \ldots, n_2 \end{aligned} \tag{7.5}$$

where $\epsilon_{1i} \sim N(0, \sigma_{\sigma_\epsilon^2})$ and $\epsilon_{2i} \sim N(0, \sigma_{\sigma_\epsilon^2})$.

Independence of X_1, X_2, ϵ_{1i}, and ϵ_{2i} is also assumed. This implies that the measurement error stems mainly from the instrument's accuracy or other technical aspects and does not actually depend on the risk of a person carrying the target disease. This justifies the assumption of equal variances for the ϵ values. In this context, Schisterman et al. (2001) [234] consider the data from a reliability study that was designed to estimate measurement error. If we denote with W_i the true biomarker score for individual i, it is assumed that:

$$w_{ij} = W_i + \epsilon_{ij} \tag{7.6}$$

for the $i-$th individual of the reliability study where $\epsilon_{ij} \sim N(0, \sigma_\epsilon^2)$. Thus,

$$\hat{\sigma}_\epsilon^2 = \frac{\sum_{i=1}^{n_1} \sum_{j=1}^{p_i} (w_{ij} - w_{i.})^2}{n_f}, \tag{7.7}$$

where $n_f = \sum_{i=1}^{n_0}(p_i - 1)$ and $w_{i.} = \sum_{j=1}^{p_i} \frac{w_{ij}}{p_i}$. If we denote with $S_1^2 = \frac{1}{n_1-1}\sum_{i=1}^{n_1}(x_{1i} - \bar{x}_2)^2$, under the assumptions stated above, an unbiased estimator of σ_1 is $\hat{\sigma}_1^2 = S_1 - \hat{\sigma}_\epsilon$. The expression of S_2 and the corresponding unbiased estimator for σ_2 are analogous. This implies an AUC estimate given by the following expression:

$$\hat{AUC} = \Phi\left(\frac{\bar{x}_2 - \bar{x}_1}{\sqrt{S_1^2 + S_2^2 - 2\hat{\sigma}_\epsilon}}\right).$$

Note that the above configuration may result in $\hat{\sigma}_1^2 < 0$ and/or $\hat{\sigma}_2^2 < 0$. Schisterman et al. (2021) [234], following the ideas of Puduri and Rao (1997) [213], recommend replacement with a very small value is such situations.

To obtain confidence intervals for the AUC, the delta method can be employed. Defining $\delta = \frac{\mu_2 - \mu_1}{\sqrt{\sigma_1^2 + \sigma_2^2}}$ we can estimate its variance by:

$$\begin{aligned} \hat{Var}(\hat{\delta}) &= \left(\frac{S_1^2}{n_1} + \frac{S_2^2}{n_2}\right) \times (S_1^2 + S_2^2 - 2\hat{\sigma}_\epsilon^2)^{-1} \\ &= \frac{(\bar{x}_2 - \bar{x}_1)^2}{4(S_1^2 + S_2^2 - 2\hat{\sigma}_\epsilon^2)^3} \times \left(\frac{2S_1^4}{n_1 - 1} + \frac{2S_2^4}{n_2 - 1} - \frac{8\hat{\sigma}_\epsilon^4}{n_f}\right). \end{aligned}$$

An approximate $(1 - a) \times 100\%$ confidence interval for δ follows:

$$\hat{\delta} \pm z_{a/2}\sqrt{\hat{Var}(\hat{\delta})},$$

which implies the following $1 - a/2$ confidence interval for the AUC:

$$\Phi\left(\hat{\delta} \pm z_{a/2}\sqrt{\hat{Var}(\hat{\delta})}\right).$$

Simulation studies have shown good coverage properties for the aforementioned confidence interval [234].

In general, using correction methods for random measurement error is often debated in the literature. The reason is the assumption that the variance of the measurement error is known or can be estimated. Non-availability of such estimates may compromise the quality of the correction. Effects of possibly heterogenous measurement error on estimated ROC curves for the binormal setting are discussed in Tosteson et al. (2005) [266].

7.4 ROC Analysis under Imperfect Reference Standard Bias

In the previous chapters, we focused only on settings where the reference standard (when available) is equivalent to a perfect test, namely, that exhibits an accuracy of 100% (sensitivity=1 and specificity=1). However, this may not always be the case.

There are several examples in the literature that involve imperfect reference standard settings. One of them refers to Alzheimer's disease, diagnosis of which is generally not definite until a neurological examination is performed in a post-mortem fashion. Due to this limitation, other imperfect tests could be employed as replacement of the reference standard, that we refer to as imperfect reference standards. When an imperfect reference standard is employed, then this might result in an under- or over-estimation of the sensitivity and specificity of the marker under study. This implies that the estimation of the ROC, as a result of biased estimation of the trade-off of the underlying sensitivities and specificities, is also going to be biased. This bias is called imperfect reference standard bias.

Another example refers to the very well-known Mantoux skin test (also known as TB skin test) that is used for the diagnosis of Tuberculosis. Pouchot et al. (1997) [215] illustrate that the Mantoux skin test, which is typically used as a reference test, is imperfect. Thus, an attempt of evaluating a new test (either a new skin test or a test of another kind) using as a reference the Mantoux might result in biased estimates of the performance of the new test under study. For additional examples that involve settings with imperfect reference standards, the interested reader is referred to Zhou et al. (2011) [314]. Therein, one can find an extensive overview of such formulations. Here, we discuss approaches that can account for the imperfect reference standard for both binary and non-binary markers.

7.4.1 Binary markers under an imperfect reference standard

Assume that classification errors for the reference standard and the test/marker under study occur independently, given the true disease status. This assumption is known as the conditional independence assumption (CIA).

Consider the configuration presented in Table 7.3 and the following notation:

$$\begin{aligned} Sens(T) &= P(T=2|D=2) \\ Sens(RS) &= P(RS=2|D=2) \\ Spec(T) &= P(T=1|D=1) \\ Spec(RS) &= P(RS=1|D=1) \\ p_{(ij)} &= P(T=i, RS=j) \end{aligned}$$

where $Sens(T)$ and $Sens(RS)$ are the sensitivities of the test and the reference standard, respectively. Similarly, with $Spec(T)$ and $Spec(RS)$, we refer to the specificities of the test and the reference standard, respectively. If we denote

TABLE 7.3
General configuration for a binary test with an imperfect reference standard.

Reference standard (RS)	Positive test result ($T = 2$)	Negative test result ($T = 1$)
RS=2	s_{22}	s_{21}
RS=1	s_{12}	s_{11}
Total	n_2	n_1

the prevalence with $\pi_D = P(D = 2)$, then it can be shown that:

$$\begin{aligned} p_{(ij)} &= \pi_D P(T = t, RS = k|D = 1) \\ &\quad +(1 - \pi_D)P(T = t, RS = k|D = 2), \quad (t, k) \in \{1, 2\}^2. \end{aligned}$$

Under the further assumption assumption of CIA, we have that:

$$P(RS, T|D) = P(RS|D)P(T|D).$$

Under the CIA, we get the following three equations:

$$\begin{aligned} p_{(22)} &= \pi_D Sens(T)Sens(RS) + (1 - \pi_D)(1 - Spec(T))(1 - Spec(RS)) \\ p_{(21)} &= \pi_D Sens(T)(1 - Sens(RS)) + (1 - \pi_D)(1 - Spec(T))(Spec(RS)) \\ p_{(12)} &= \pi_D(1 - Sens(T))Sens(RS) + (1 - \pi_D)(Spec(T))(1 - Spec(RS)) \end{aligned}$$

which involve five parameters to be estimated, namely, π_D, $Sens(T)$, $Spec(T)$, $Sens(RS)$, and $Spec(RS)$. Hence, there is an issue of identifiability since we have three equations with five parameters. Additional assumptions will restrict this system more and thus could make modeling identifiable. Such assumptions could involve one of the following: (i) $Sens(RS)$ and $Spec(RS)$ are known, (ii) $Sens(RS) = Sens(T) = 1$, (iii) $Spec(RS) = Spec(T) = 1$. Assuming the first statement, the resulting likelihood is of the form:

$$\begin{aligned} L &= (Sens(RS)Sens(T)\pi_D + (1 - Spec(RS))(1 - Spec(T))(1 - \pi_D))^{s_{22}} \\ &\times (Sens(RS)(1 - Sens(T))\pi_D + (1 - Spec(RS))Spec(T)(1 - \pi_D))^{s_{21}} \\ &\times ((1 - Sens(RS))Sens(T)\pi_D + Spec(RS)(1 - Spec(T))(1 - \pi_D))^{s_{12}} \\ &\times ((1 - Sens(RS))(1 - Sens(T))\pi_D + (Spec(RS))(Spec(T))(1 - \pi_D))^{s_{11}} \end{aligned}$$

and the resulting maximum likelihood estimates can be found in closed form and are given by:

$$\hat{Sens}(T) = \frac{Spec(RS)(s_{22}+s_{12})-s_{12}}{(n_1+n_2)Spec(RS)-(s_{12}+s_{11})}$$

$$\hat{Spec}(T) = \frac{Sens(RS)(s_{21}+s_{11})-s_{21}}{(n_1+n_2)Sens(RS)-(s_{22}+s_{21})}$$

$$\hat{\pi} = \frac{(n_1+n_2)Spec(RS)-(s_{12}+s_{11})}{n_1+n_2}$$

These estimates are the corrected versions of the sensitivity and specificity under an imperfect reference standard and the assumptions discussed above. Other approaches that are discussed in Dendukuri and Joseph (2001) [65] and Zhou et al. (2011) [314] involve a Bayesian framework that assumes conjugate beta priors for the aforementioned five parameters. In such a framework, the likelihood has a complicated form and for the posterior distribution Joseph et al. (1995) [135] consider the Gibbs sampler. We refer the interested reader to their paper for the computational details.

7.4.2 Non-binary markers under an imperfect reference standard

The literature involving non-binary biomarkers under an imperfect reference standard setting is limited. This is also highlighted in Hui and Zhou (1998) [130]. One paper that deals with ROC estimation but has raised some concerns is that of Henkelman et al. (1990) [120]. They propose a maximum likelihood approach using a multivariate normal mixture latent model. Begg and Metz (1990) [30] discuss various limitations of this approach, and they recommend that further research needs to be done before one could use this method in practice. Here, we discuss the method of Zhou et al. (2005) [311] which generalizes the concept to the presence of K available ordinal tests. Note that, we still need the conditional independence assumption.

Let $Y_1, Y_2, \ldots, Y_K$ be random variables that correspond to the measurements of K different *ordinal* tests that are all applied on the same patient. The corresponding TPR and FPR are then:

$$TPR_k(j) = P(Y_k \geq j | D = 2)$$
$$FPR_k(j) = P(Y_k \geq j | D = 1)$$

where $j = 1, 2, \ldots, J+1$. The nonparametric ROC estimate is a discrete function defined by the pairs $(FPR_k(j), TPR_k(j))$, $j = 1, 2, \ldots, J+1$. The

ROC is then drawn by simply connecting the coordinates of these FPR and TPR pairs. Under this configuration, the AUC is given by:

$$\begin{aligned} AUC_k &= \sum_{j=1}^{J-1} \left(P(Y_k = j|D = 1) \sum_{l=j+1}^{J} P(Y_k = l|D = 2) \right) \\ &+ \frac{1}{2} \sum_{j=1}^{J} P(Y_k = j|D = 1) P(Y_k = j|D = 2). \end{aligned}$$

For the technical details about the formulation of the likelihood and its maximization, we refer to the work of Zhou et al. (2005) [311]. Therein, the authors also describe the EM algorithm for the case where the marker measurements are not ordinal but follow a normal distribution. This version of the EM algorithm is implemented by a modification of the ROCFIT program [172]. Once we obtain the underlying parameter estimates, the ROC curve and its AUC can be obtained.

Further topics regarding the imperfect reference standard concept involve multiple binary tests, as well as relaxing the conditional independence assumption [314].

7.5 Exercises

7.1 Provide a different numerical example changing the numbers in Table 7.2 and using the estimates in Section 7.1.1.

7.2 Obtain VUS values and confidence intervals for the IPW and SPE methods described in Section 7.1.3.1 using the package `bcROCsurface`.

7.3 Construct a numerical example for the procedures described in Section 7.4.1.

Bibliography

[1] A.G. Abraham, D.D. Duncan, S.J. Gange, and S. West. Computer-aided assessment of diagnostic images for epidemiological research. *BMC Medical Research Methodology*, 9(1):art. no. 74, 2009.

[2] K.A. Aho. *Foundational and Applied Statistics for Biologists Using R*. CRC Press, 2013.

[3] M.G. Akritas. Nearest neighbor estimation of a bivariate distribution under random censoring. *The Annals of Statistics*, 22(3):1299–1327, 1994.

[4] T.A. Alonzo and C.T. Nakas. Comparison of roc umbrella volumes with an application to the assessment of lung cancer diagnostic markers. *Biometrical Journal*, 49(5):654–664, 2007.

[5] T.A. Alonzo, C.T. Nakas, C.T. Yiannoutsos, and S. Bucher. A comparison of tests for restricted orderings in the three-class case. *Statistics in Medicine*, 28(7):1144–1158, 2009.

[6] T.A. Alonzo and M.S. Pepe. Assessing accuracy of a continuous screening test in the presence of verification bias. *Journal of the Royal Statistical Society: Series C (Applied Statistics)*, 54(1):173–190, 2005.

[7] W.N. Arifin and U.K. Yusof. Correcting for partial verification bias in diagnostic accuracy studies: A tutorial using R. *Statistics in Medicine*, 41(9):1709–1727, 2022.

[8] J.N. Arvesen. Jackknifing U-statistics. *Annals of Mathematical Statistics*, 40:2076–2100, 1969.

[9] T. Augustin and F.P.A. Coolen. Nonparametric predictive inference and interval probability. *Journal of Statistical Planning and Inference*, 124:251–272, 2004.

[10] D. Bamber. The area above the ordinal dominance graph and the area below the receiver operating characteristic graph. *Journal of Mathematical Psychology*, 12(4):387–415, 1975.

[11] A. Bandos and N. Obuchowski. Evaluation of diagnostic accuracy in free-response detection-localization tasks using ROC tools. *Statistical Methods in Medical Research*, 28:1808–1825, 2019.

[12] A.I. Bandos, B. Guo, and D. Gur. Estimating the area under ROC curve when the fitted binormal curves demonstrate improper shape. *Academic Radiology*, 24:209–219, 2017.

[13] A.I. Bandos, H. Rockette, T. Song, and D. Gur. Area under the free-response ROC curve (FROC) and a related summary index. *Biometrics*, 65:247–256, 2009.

[14] A.I. Bandos, H.E. Rockette, and D. Gur. A permutation test sensitive to differences in areas for comparing ROC curves from a paired setting. *Statistics in Medicine*, 24:2873–2893, 2005.

[15] L. Bantis, C.T. Nakas, B. Reiser, D. Myall, and J.C. Dalrymple-Alford. Construction of joint confidence regions for the optimal true class fractions of receiver operating characteristic (ROC) surfaces and manifolds. *Statistical Methods in Medical Research*, 26:1429–1442, 2017.

[16] L.E. Bantis, C.T. Nakas, and B. Reiser. Construction of confidence regions in the ROC space after the estimation of the optimal youden index-based cut-off point. *Biometrics*, 70:212–223, 2014.

[17] L.E. Bantis, C.T. Nakas, and B. Reiser. Construction of confidence intervals for the maximum of the youden index and the corresponding cutoff point of a continuous biomarker. *Biometrical Journal*, 61:138–156, 2019.

[18] L.E. Bantis, C.T. Nakas, and B. Reiser. Statistical inference for the difference between two maximized youden indices obtained from correlated biomarkers. *Biometrical Journal*, 63:1241–1253, 2021.

[19] L.E. Bantis and J.V. Tsimikas. On optimal biomarker cutoffs accounting for misclassification costs in diagnostic trilemmas with applications to pancreatic cancer. *Statistics in Medicine*, 41(18):3527–3546, 2022.

[20] L.E. Bantis, J.V. Tsimikas, G.R. Chambers, M. Capello, S. Hanash, and Z. Feng. The length of the receiver operating characteristic curve and the two cutoff youden index within a robust framework for discovery, evaluation, and cutoff estimation in biomarker studies involving improper receiver operating characteristic curves. *Statistics in Medicine*, 40:1767–1789, 2021.

[21] L.E. Bantis, J.V. Tsimikas, and S.D. Georgiou. Survival estimation through the cumulative hazard function with monotone natural cubic splines. *Lifetime Data Analysis*, 18(3):364–396, 2012.

[22] L.E. Bantis, J.V. Tsimikas, and S.D. Georgiou. Smooth ROC curves and surfaces for markers subject to a limit of detection using monotone natural cubic splines. *Biometrical Journal*, 55(5):719–740, 2013.

[23] L.E. Bantis, J.V. Tsimikas, and S.D. Georgiou. Survival estimation through the cumulative hazard with monotone natural cubic splines using convex optimization-the HCNS approach. *Computer Methods and Programs in Biomedicine*, 190:105357, 2020.

[24] L.E. Bantis, Q. Yan, J.V. Tsimikas, and Z. Feng. Estimation of smooth ROC curves for biomarkers with limits of detection. *Statistics in Medicine*, 36(24):3830–3843, 2017.

[25] L.E. Bantis and Feng Z. Comparison of two correlated ROC curves at a given specificity level. *Statistics in Medicine*, 35(24):4352–4367, 2016.

[26] L.E. Bantis and Feng Z. Comparison of two correlated roc surfaces at a given pair of true classification rates. *Statistics in Medicine*, 37(27):4022–4035, 2018.

[27] V.T. Bazylev. *'Hypersurface' in Encyclopedia of Mathematics.* Kluwer Academic Publishers, 2002.

[28] C. Beam, P. Layde, and D. Sullivan. Variability in the interpretation of screening mammogram. *Archives of Internal Medicine*, 156:209–213, 1996.

[29] C.B. Begg and R.A. Greenes. Assessment of diagnostic tests when disease verification is subject to selection bias. *Biometrics*, 39:207–215, 1983.

[30] C.B. Begg and C.E. Metz. Consensus diagnosis and gold standards. *Medical Decision Making*, 10:29–30, 1990.

[31] S. Beiden, R. Wagner, and G. Campbell. Components-of-variance models and multiple-bootstrap experiments: An alternative method for random-effects, receiver operating characteristic analysis. *Academic Radiology*, 7:341–349, 2000.

[32] Z.W. Birnbaum and O.M. Klose. Bounds for the variance of the mann-whitney statistic. *Annals of Mathematical Statistics*, 28:933–945, 1957.

[33] W.C. Blackwelder. "proving the null hypothesis" in clinical trials. *Controlled Clinical Trials*, 3:345–353, 1982.

[34] J.M. Bland. *An Introduction to Medical Statistics*, 4th edition. OUP Oxford, 2015.

[35] J.D. Blume. Bounding sample size projections for the area under a ROC curve. *Journal of Statistical Planning and Inference*, 139:711–721, 2009.

[36] G.E.P. Box and D.R. Cox. An analysis of transformations. *Journal of the Royal Statistical Society. Series B (Methodological)*, 26:211–252, 1964.

[37] K. Boyd. Area under the precision-recall curve: Point estimates and confidence intervals. *Machine Learning and Knowledge Discovery in Databases*, 8190:451–466, 2013.

[38] K. Boyd, V. Santos Costa, J. Davis, and D.C. Page. Unachievable region in precision-recall space and its effect on empirical evaluation. *Proceedings of the 29th International Conference on Machine Learning*, Edinburgh, Scotland, UK:349–355, 2012.

[39] A.J. Branscum, W.O. Johnson, T.E. Hanson, and I.A. Gardner. Bayesian semiparametric ROC curve estimation and disease diagnosis. *Statistics in Medicine*, 27:2474–2496, 2008.

[40] T.M. Braun and T.A. Alonzo. A modified sign test for comparing paired roc curves. *Biostatistics*, 9:364–372, 2008.

[41] L.D. Brown, T. Cai, and A. Das Gupta. Interval estimation for a binomial proportion. *Statistical Science*, 16:101–133, 2001.

[42] R. Bruña, J. Poza, C. Gòmez, M. García, A. Fernández, and R. Hornero. Analysis of spontaneous meg activity in mild cognitive impairment and alzheimer's disease using spectral entropies and statistical complexity measures. *Journal of Neural Engineering*, 9(3):art. no. 036007, 2012.

[43] L.C. Brumback, M.S. Pepe, and T.A. Alonzo. Using the ROC curve for gauging treatment effect in clinical trials. *Statistics in Medicine*, 25(4):575–590, 2006.

[44] M. Buckland and F. Grey. The relationship between recall and precision. *Journal of the American Society for Information Science*, 45:12–19, 1994.

[45] T. Cai. Semi-parametric roc regression analysis with placement values. *Biostatistics*, 5(1):45–60, 2004.

[46] T. Cai, M.S. Pepe, Y. Zheng, T. Lumley, and N.S. Jenny. The sensitivity and specificity of markers for event times. *Biostatistics*, 7(2):182–197, 2006.

[47] G. Campbell and M.V. Ratnaparkhi. An application of lomax distributions in receiver operating characteristic (ROC) curve analysis. *Communications in Statistics – Theory and Methods*, 22:1681–1697, 1993.

[48] C. Carraccio, K. Blotny, and M.C. Fisher. Cerebrospinal fluid analysis in systematically ill children without central nervous system disease. *Pediatrics*, 96:48–51, 1995.

[49] M.P. Cecil, A.S. Kosinski, M.T. Jones, A. Taylor, N.P. Alazraki, R.I. Pettigrew, and W.S. Weintraub. The importance of work-up (verification) bias correction in assessing the accuracy of spect thallium-201

testing for the diagnosis of coronary artery disease. *Journal of Clinical Epidemiology*, 49(7):735–742, 1996.

[50] D.P. Chakraborty and K.S. Berbaum. Observer studies involving detection and localization: Modeling, analysis, and validation. *Medical Physics*, 31:2313–2330, 2004.

[51] A. Cianferoni, J.P. Garrett, D.R. Naimi, K. Khullar, and J.M. Spergel. Predictive values for food challenge-induced severe reactions: Development of a simple food challenge score. *Israel Medical Association Journal*, 14(1):24–28, 2012.

[52] S. Clémençon, S. Robbiano, and N. Vayatis. Ranking data with ordinal labels: Optimality and pairwise aggregation. *Machine Learning*, 91(1):67–104, 2013.

[53] M. Coffin and S. Sukhatme. Receiver operating characteristic studies and measurement errors. *Biometrics*, 53:823–837, 1997.

[54] D.J. Coleman, R.H. Silverman, M.J. Rondeau, H.O. Lloyd, A.A. Khanifar, and R.V.P. Chan. Age-related macular degeneration: Choroidal ischaemia? *British Journal of Opthalmology*, 97(8):1020–1023, 2013.

[55] J. Cook and V. Ramadas. When to consult precision-recall curves. *The Stata Journal*, 20:131–148, 2020.

[56] N.R. Cook. Quantifying the added value of new biomarkers: How and how not. *Diagnostic and Prognostic Research*, 2:14, 2018.

[57] T. Coolen-Maturi, P. Coolen-Schrijner, and F.P.A. Coolen. Nonparametric predictive inference for binary diagnostic tests. *Journal of Statistical Theory and Practice*, 6:665–680, 2012.

[58] T. Coolen-Maturi, F.F. Elkhafifi, and F.P.A. Coolen. Nonparametric predictive inference for three-group ROC analysis, technical report no 1307, department of mathematical sciences, university of durham, uk, https://npi-statistics.com/pdfs/papers/CoEC2013.pdf, 2013.

[59] R.B. D'Agostino, J.M. Massaro, and L.M. Sullivan. Non-inferiority trials: Design concepts and issues – the encounters of academic consultants in statistics. *Statistics in Medicine*, 22:169–186, 2003.

[60] J.C. Dalrymple-Alford, M.R. MacAskill, C.T. Nakas, L. Livingston, C. Graham, G.P. Crucian, T.R. Melzer, J. Kirwan, R. Keenan, S. Wells, R.J. Porter, R. Watts, and T.J. Anderson. The moca: Well suited screen for cognitive impairment in parkinson disease. *Neurology*, 75(19):1717–1725, 2010.

[61] O. Davidov and A. Herman. Ordinal dominance curve based inference for stochastically ordered distributions. *Journal of the Royal Statistical Society. Series B: Statistical Methodology*, 74(5):825–847, 2012.

[62] J. Davis and M. Goadrich. The relationship between precision-recall and roc curves. *Proceedings of the 23rd International Conference on Machine Learning*, New York, USA:233–240, 2006.

[63] A.C. Davison and D.V. Hinkley. *Bootstrap Methods and Their Application*. Cambridge University Press, 1997.

[64] E.R. DeLong, D.M. DeLong, and D.L. Clarke-Pearson. Comparing the areas under two or more correlated receiver operating characteristic curves: A nonparameteric approach. *Biometrics*, 44:837–845, 1988.

[65] N. Dendukuri and L. Joseph. Bayesian approaches to modeling the conditional dependence between diagnostic tests. *Biometrics*, 44:837–845, 2001.

[66] S. Díaz-Coto, P. Martínez-Camblor, and S. Pérez-Fernández. smoothroctime: An R package for time-dependent ROC curve estimation. *Computational Statistics*, 35:1231–1251, 2020.

[67] L.E. Dodd and M.S. Pepe. Partial AUC estimation and regression. *Biometrics*, 59:614–623, 2003.

[68] D.D. Dorfman and E. Alf. Maximum likelihood estimation of parameters of signal detection theory – a direct solution. *Psychometrika*, 33:117–124, 1968.

[69] D.D. Dorfman and E. Alf. Maximum-likelihood estimation of parameters of signal-detection theory and determination of confidence intervals – rating-method data. *Journal of Mathematical Psychology*, 6:487–496, 1969.

[70] D.D. Dorfman, K.S. Berbaum, and R.V. Lenth. Multireader, multicase receiver operating characteristic methodology: A bootstrap analysis. *Academic Radiology*, 2:626–633, 1995.

[71] D.D. Dorfman, K.S. Berbaum, and C.E. Metz. Receiver operating characteristic rating analysis: Generalization to the population of readers and patients with the jackknife method. *Investigative Radiology*, 27:723–731, 1992.

[72] D.D. Dorfman, K.S. Berbaum, C.E. Metz, R.V. Lenth, J.A. Hanley, and H. Abu Dagga. Proper receiver operating characteristic analysis: The bigamma model. *Academic Radiology*, 4:138–149, 1997.

[73] S. Dreiseitl, L. Ohno-Machado, and M. Binder. Comparing three-class diagnostic tests by three-way ROC analysis. *Medical Decision Making*, 20:323–331, 2000.

[74] A. Dunngalvin, D. Daly, C. Cullinane, E. Stenke, D. Keeton, M. Erlewyn-Lajeunesse, G.C. Roberts, J. Lucas, and J.O. Hourihane. Highly accurate prediction of food challenge outcome using routinely available clinical data. *Journal of Allergy and Clinical Immunology*, 127(3):633–639, 2011.

[75] D.C. Edwards. Validation of monte carlo estimates of three-class ideal observer operating points for normal data. *Academic Radiology*, 20(7):908–914, 2013.

[76] D.C. Edwards and C.E. Metz. Optimization of restricted roc surfaces in three-class classification tasks. *IEEE Transactions on Medical Imaging*, 26(10):1345–1356, 2007.

[77] D.C. Edwards and C.E. Metz. The three-class ideal observer for univariate normal data: Decision variable and ROC surface properties. *Journal of Mathematical Psychology*, 56(4):256–273, 2012.

[78] S. Eguchi and J. Copas. A class of logistic-type discriminant functions. *Biometrika*, 89:1–22, 2002.

[79] W.L. England. An exponential model used for optimal threshold selection on roc curves. *Medical Decision Making*, 8:120–131, 1988.

[80] R. Etzioni, M. Pepe, G. Longton, C. Hu, and G. Goodman. Incorporating the time dimension in receiver operating characteristic curves: A case study of prostate cancer. *Medical Decision Making*, 19(3):242–251, 1999.

[81] R.M. Everson and J.E. Fieldsend. Multi-class roc analysis from a multi-objective optimisation perspective. *Pattern Recognition Letters*, 27(8):918–927, 2006.

[82] D. Faraggi. The effect of random measurement error on receiver operating characteristic (ROC) curves. *Statistics in Medicine*, 19:61–70, 2000.

[83] D. Faraggi. Adjusting receiver operating curves and related indices for covariates. *Journal of the Royal Statistical Society Series D*, 52:179–192, 2003.

[84] D. Faraggi and B. Reiser. Estimation of the area under the ROC curve. *Statistics in Medicine*, 21:3093–3106, 2002.

[85] Y. Feng and L. Tian. Measuring diagnostic accuracy for biomarkers under tree-ordering. *Statistical Methods in Medical Research*, 28:1328–1346, 2018.

[86] Y. Feng and L. Tian. Flexible diagnostic measures and new cut-point selection methods under multiple ordered classes. *Pharmaceutical Statistics*, 21(1):220–240, 2022.

[87] R. Fluss, D. Faraggi, and B. Reiser. Estimation of the youden index and its associated cutoff point. *Biometrical Journal*, 47:458–472, 2005.

[88] A.M. Franco-Pereira, C.T. Nakas, A.B. Leichtle, and M.C. Pardo. Bootstrap-based testing approaches for the assessment of the diagnostic accuracy of biomarkers subject to a limit of detection. *Statistical Methods in Medical Research*, 28(5):1564–1578, 2019.

[89] A.M. Franco-Pereira, C.T. Nakas, and M.C. Pardo. Biomarker assessment in roc curve analysis using the length of the curve as an index of diagnostic accuracy: The binormal model framework. *AStA Advances in Statistical Analysis*, 104:625–647, 2020.

[90] M.H. Gail and S.B. Green. A generalization of the one-sided two-sample kolmogorov-smirnov statistic for evaluating diagnostic tests. *Biometrics*, 32:561–570, 1976.

[91] B.D. Gallas, A. Bandos, F.W. Samuelson, and R.F. Wagner. A framework for random-effects ROC analysis: Biases with the bootstrap and other variance estimators. *Communications in Statistics – Theory and Methods*, 38(15):2586–2603, 2009.

[92] Y. Gao and L. Tian. Confidence interval estimation for sensitivity and difference between two sensitivities at a given specificity under tree ordering. *Statistics in Medicine*, 40:3695–3723, 2021.

[93] C.A. Gatsonis. Random-effects models for diagnostic accuracy data. *Academic Radiology*, 2 Suppl 1:S14–21; discussion S57–67, S61–4 pa, 1995.

[94] C.A. Gatsonis. Receiver operating characteristic analysis for the evaluation of diagnosis and prediction. *Radiology*, 253(3):593–596, 2009.

[95] D. Ghosh. Incorporating monotonicity into the evaluation of a biomarker. *Biostatistics*, 8:402–413, 2007.

[96] M. Gönen and G. Heller. Lehmann family of roc curves. *Medical Decision Making*, 30:509–517, 2010.

[97] J. Grau, I. Grosse, and J. Keilwagen. PRROC: Computing and visualizing precision-recall and receiver operating characteristic curves in R. *Bioinformatics*, 31:2595–2597, 2015.

[98] M. Greiner, D. Pfeiffer, and R.D. Smith. Principles and practical applications of the receiver-operating characteristic analysis for diagnostic tests. *Preventive Veterinary Medicine*, 45:23–41, 2000.

[99] P. Guangming, W. Xiping, and Z. Wang. Nonparametric statistical inference for $p(x < y < z)$. *Sankhya A: The Indian Journal of Statistics*, 75(1):118–138, 2013.

[100] D.G. Haider, T. Klemenz, G.M. Fiedler, C.T. Nakas, A.K. Exadaktylos, and A.B. Leichtle. High sensitive cardiac troponin T: Testing the test. *International Journal of Cardiology*, 228:779–783, 2017.

[101] P. Hall, R.J. Hyndman, and Y. Fan. Nonparametric confidence intervals for receiver operating characteristic curves. *Biometrika*, 91:743–750, 2004.

[102] Y. Han, P.S. Albert, C.D. Berg, N. Wentzensen, H.A. Katki, and D. Liu. Statistical approaches using longitudinal biomarkers for disease early detection: A comparison of methodologies. *Statistics in Medicine*, 39:4405–4420, 2020.

[103] D.J. Hand and R.J. Till. A simple generalisation of the area under the roc curve for multiple-class classification problems. *Machine Learning*, 45:171–186, 2001.

[104] J.A. Hanley. The use of the binormal model for parametric roc analysis of quantitative diagnostic tests. *Statistics in Medicine*, 15:1575–1585, 1996.

[105] J.A. Hanley and B.J. McNeil. The meaning and use of the area under a receiver operating characteristic (ROC) curve. *Radiology*, 143:29–36, 1982.

[106] T.E. Hanson, A. Kottas, and A.J. Branscum. Modelling stochastic order in the analysis of receiver operating characteristic data: Bayesian nonparametric approaches. *Journal of the Royal Statistical Society: Series C*, 57:207–225, 2008.

[107] O. Harel and X.H. Zhou. Multiple imputation for correcting verification bias. *Statistics in Medicine*, 25(22):3769–3786, 2006.

[108] O. Harel and X.H. Zhou. Rejoinder to multiple imputation for correcting verification bias. *Statistics in Medicine*, 26(15):3047–3050, 2007.

[109] F.E. Harrell, K.L. Lee, and D.B. Mark. Multivariable prognostic models: Issues in developing models, evaluating assumptions and adequacy, and measuring and reducing errors. *Statistics in Medicine*, 15:361–387, 1996.

[110] H. He, J.M. Lyness, and M.P. McDermott. Direct estimation of the area under the receiver operating characteristic curve in the presence of verification bias. *Statistics in Medicine*, 28(3):361–376, 2009.

[111] X. He and E.C. Frey. Three-class roc analysis - the equal error utility assumption and the optimality of three-class ROC surface using the ideal observer. *IEEE Transactions on Medical Imaging*, 25(8):979–986, 2006.

[112] X. He and E.C. Frey. The meaning and use of the volume under a three-class ROC surface (vus). *IEEE Transactions on Medical Imaging*, 27(5):577–588, 2008.

[113] X. He and E.C. Frey. The validity of three-class hotelling trace (3-ht) in describing three-class task performance: Comparison of three-class volume under ROC surface (vus) and 3-ht. *IEEE Transactions on Medical Imaging*, 28(2):185–193, 2009.

[114] X. He, B.D. Gallas, and E.C. Frey. Three-class ROC analysis: Toward a general decision theoretic solution. *IEEE Transactions on Medical Imaging*, 29(1):206–215, 2010.

[115] X. He, C.E. Metz, B.M.W. Tsui, J.M. Links, and E.C. Frey. Three-class ROC analysis - a decision theoretic approach under the ideal observer framework. *IEEE Transactions on Medical Imaging*, 25(5):571–581, 2006.

[116] P.J. Heagerty, T. Lumley, and M.S. Pepe. Time-dependent roc curves for censored survival data and a diagnostic marker. *Biometrics*, 56(2):337–344, 2000.

[117] P.J. Heagerty and Y. Zheng. Survival model predictive accuracy and ROC curves. *Biometrics*, 61(1):92–105, 2005.

[118] P.S. Heckerling. Parametric three-way receiver operating characteristic surface analysis using mathematica. *Medical Decision Making*, 21:409–417, 2001.

[119] G. Heller, V.E. Seshan, C.S. Moskowitz, and M. Gönen. Inference for the difference in the area under the ROC curve derived from nested binary regression models. *Biostatistics*, 18:260–274, 2017.

[120] R.M. Henkelman, I. Kay, and M.J. Bronskill. Receiver operator characteristic (ROC) analysis without truth. *Medical Decision Making*, 7:354–370, 1990.

[121] J. Hilden. The area under the ROC curve and its competitors. *Medical Decision Making*, 11:95–101, 1991.

[122] S.L. Hillis and K.M. Schartz. Multireader sample size program for diagnostic studies: Demonstration and methodology. *Journal of Medical Imaging*, 5:045503, 2018.

[123] W. Hoeffding. A class of statistics with asymptotically normal distribution. *Annals of Mathematical Statistics*, 19:293–325, 1948.

[124] R.W. Hornung and L.D. Reed. Estimation of average concentration in the presence of nondetectable values. *Applied Occupational and Environmental Hygiene*, 5:46–51, 1990.

[125] D.G. Horvitz and D.J. Thompson. A generalization of sampling without replacement from a finite universe. *Journal of the American statistical Association*, 47(260):663–685, 1952.

[126] D.W. Hosmer, S. Lemeshow, and R.X. Sturdivant. *Applied Logistic Regression,* 3rd edition. Wiley, 2013.

[127] F. Hsieh and B.W. Turnbull. Nonparametric and semiparametric estimation of the receiver operating characteristic curve. *Annals of Statistics*, 24(1):25–40, 1996.

[128] J. Hua and L. Tian. A comprehensive and comparative review of optimal cut-points selection methods for diseases with multiple ordinal stages. *Journal of Biopharmaceutical Statistics*, 30(1):46–68, 2020.

[129] J. Hua and L. Tian. Combining multiple biomarkers to linearly maximize the diagnostic accuracy under ordered multi-class setting. *Statistical Methods in Medical Research*, 30:1101–1118, 2021.

[130] S.L. Hui and X.H. Zhou. Evaluation of diagnostic tests without gold standards. *Statistical Methods in Medical Research*, 7:354–370, 1998.

[131] V. Inácio, A.A. Turkman, C.T. Nakas, and T.A. Alonzo. Nonparametric bayesian estimation of the three-way receiver operating characteristic surface. *Biometrical Journal*, 53(6):1011–1024, 2011.

[132] V. Inácio de Carvalho and A.J. Brunscam. Bayesian nonparametric inference for the three-class youden index and its associated optimal cutoff points. *Statistical Methods in Medical Research*, 27(3):689–700, 2018.

[133] V. Inácio de Carvalho, A. Jara, T.E. Hanson, and M. de Carvalho. Bayesian nonparametric roc regression modeling. *Bayesian Analysis*, 8(3):623–646, 2013.

[134] H. Ishwaran and C.A. Gatsonis. A general class of hierarchical ordinal regression models with applications to correlated ROC analysis. *The Canadian Journal of Statistics*, 28(4):731–750, 2000.

[135] L. Joseph, T.W. Gyorkos, and L. Coupal. Bayesian estimation of disease prevalence and the parameters of diagnostic tests in the absence of a gold standard. *American Journal of Epidemiology*, 3:263–272, 1995.

[136] L. Kang and L. Tian. Estimation of the volume under the roc surface with three ordinal diagnostic categories. *Computational Statistics and Data Analysis*, 62:39–51, 2013.

[137] J. Keilwagen, I. Grosse, and J. Grau. Area under precision-recall curves for weighted and unweighted data. *PLoS ONE*, 9:e92209, 2014.

[138] G.J. Kelloff, J.M. Hoffman, B. Johnson, H.I. Scher, B.A. Siegel, E.Y. Cheng, B.D. Cheson, J. O'Shaughnessy, K.Z. Guyton, D.A. Mankoff, L. Shankar, S.M. Larson, C.C. Sigman, R.L. Schilsky, and D.C. Sullivan. Progress and promise of fdg-pet imaging for cancer patient management and oncologic drug development. *Clinical Cancer Research*, 15(11):2785–2808, 2005.

[139] C. Kooperberg and C.J. Stone. Logspline density estimation for censored data. *Journal of Computational and Graphical Statistics*, 1:301–328, 1992.

[140] A.S. Kosinski and H.X. Barnhart. Accounting for nonignorable verification bias in assessment of diagnostic tests. *Biometrics*, 59(1):163–171, 2003.

[141] A.S. Kosinski and H.X. Barnhart. A global sensitivity analysis of performance of a medical diagnostic test when verification bias is present. *Statistics in Medicine*, 22(17):2711–2721, 2003.

[142] A.S. Kosinski, Y. Chen, and R.H. Lyles. Sample size calculations for evaluating a diagnostic test when the gold standard is missing at random. *Statistics in Medicine*, 29:1572–1579, 2010.

[143] W.J. Krzanowski and D.J. Hand. *ROC Curves for Continuous Data.* CRC Press, 2009.

[144] W.J. Krzanowski and D.J. Hand. Testing the difference between two kolmogorov-smirnov values in the context of receiver operating characteristic curves. *Journal of Applied Statistics*, 38:437–450, 2011.

[145] E.L. Lehmann. *Nonparametrics: Statistical Methods Based on Ranks.* Springer, 2006.

[146] A. Leichtle, U. Ceglarek, P. Weinert, C.T. Nakas, J.M. Nuoffer, J. Kase, T. Conrad, H. Witzigmann, J. Thiery, and G. Fiedler. Pancreatic carcinoma, pancreatitis, and healthy controls: Metabolite models in a three-class diagnostic dilemma. *Metabolomics*, 9(3):677–687, 2013.

[147] C. Lesmeister. *Mastering Machine Learning with R,* 3rd edition. Packt publishing, 2019.

[148] C.R. Li, C.T. Liao, and J.P. Liu. A non-inferiority test for diagnostic accuracy based on the paired partial areas under ROC curves. *Statistics in Medicine*, 27:1762–1776, 2008.

[149] J. Li and J. Fine. ROC analysis with multiple classes and multiple tests: Methodology and its application in microarray studies. *Biostatistics*, 9:566–576, 2008.

[150] J. Li and X.H. Zhou. Nonparametric and semiparametric estimation of the three-way receiver operating characteristic surface. *Journal of Statistical Planning and Inference*, 139(12):4133–4142, 2009.

[151] J.L. Li, X.H. Zhou, and J.P. Fine. A regression approach to roc surface, with applications to alzheimer's disease. *Science China Mathematics*, 55(8):1583–1595, 2012.

[152] R.J.A. Little and D.B. Rubin. *Statistical Analysis with Missing Data*, 3rd edition. John Wiley & Sons, 2019.

[153] J.P. Liu, M.C. Ma, C.Y Wu, and J.Y. Tai. Tests of equivalence and non-inferiority for diagnostic accuracy based on the paired areas under ROC curves. *Statistics in Medicine*, 25:1219–1238, 2006.

[154] S. Liu, J. Yang, X. Zeng, H. Song, J. Cen, and X. Weichao. An efficient and user-friendly software tool for ordered multi-class receiver operating characteristic analysis based on python. *SoftwareX*, 19(101175), 2022.

[155] X. Liu. Classification accuracy and cut point selection. *Statistics in Medicine*, 31:2676–2686, 2012.

[156] C.J. Lloyd. Using smooth receiver operating characteristic curves to summarize and compare diagnostic systems. *Journal of the American Statistical Association*, 93:1356–1364, 1998.

[157] C.J. Lloyd and Z. Yong. Kernel estimators of the roc curve are better than empirical. *Statistics & Probability Letters*, 44:221–228, 1999.

[158] Y. Lu, H. Jin, and H.K. Genant. On the non-inferiority of a diagnostic test based on paired observations. *Statistics in Medicine*, 22:3029–3044, 2003.

[159] J. Luo and C. Xiong. Youden index and associated cut-points for three ordinal diagnostic groups. *Communications in Statistics – Simulation and Computation*, 42(6):1213–1234, 2013.

[160] G. Ma and W.J. Hall. Confidence bands for receiver operating characteristic curves. *Medical Decision Making*, 13:191–197, 1993.

[161] S. Ma and J. Huang. Combining multiple markers for classification using ROC. *Biometrics*, 63:751–757, 2007.

[162] E.Z. Martinez, J.A. Achcar, and F. Louzada-Neto. Estimators of sensitivity and specificity in the presence of verification bias: A bayesian approach. *Computational Statistics and Data Analysis*, 51(2):601–611, 2006.

[163] P. Martínez-Camblor, N. Corral, C. Rey, J. Pascual, and E. Cernuda-Morollón. Receiver operating characteristic curve generalization for non-monotone relationships. *Statistical Methods in Medical Research*, 26:113–123, 2017.

[164] P. Martínez-Camblor and J.C. Pardo-Fernández. Parametric estimates for the receiver operating characteristic curve generalization for non-monotone relationships. *Statistical Methods in Medical Research*, 28:2032–2048, 2019.

[165] S. Matsui, M. Buyse, and R. Simon. *Design and Analysis of Clinical trials for Predictive Medicine.* CRC Press, 2015.

[166] D.K. McClish. Analyzing a portion of the ROC curve. *Medical Decision Making*, 9:190–195, 1989.

[167] D.K. McClish. Evaluation of the accuracy of medical tests in a region around the optimal point. *Academic Radiology*, 19:1484–1490, 2012.

[168] P. McCullagh. Regression models for ordinal data. *Journal of the Royal Statistical Society, Series B*, 42:109–142, 1980.

[169] M.W. McIntosh and M.S. Pepe. Combining several screening tests: Optimality of the risk score. *Biometrics*, 58:657–664, 2002.

[170] C.E. Metz, B.A. Herman, and J.H. Shen. Maximum likelihood estimation of receiver operating characteristic (ROC) curves from continuously-distributed data. *Statistics in Medicine*, 17:1033–1053, 1998.

[171] C.E. Metz and H.B. Kronman. Statistical significance tests for binormal ROC curves. *Journal of Mathematical Psychology*, 22:218–243, 1980.

[172] C.E. Metz, J.H. Shen, P.L. Wang, and H.B. Kronman. ROCFIT software. *Technical Report, University of Chicago*, 1994.

[173] C.E. Metz, P.L. Wang, and H.B. Kronman. Information processing in medical imaging. *Proceedings of the 8th Conference, Brussels, 29 August - 2 September 1983.* Kluwer, 1984.

[174] G. Migliaretti, P. Ciaramitaro, P. Berchialla, C. Scarinzi, R. Andrini, A. Orlando, and G. Faccani. Teleconsulting for minor head injury: The piedmont experience. *Journal of Telemedicine and Telecare*, 19(1):33–35, 2013.

[175] A. Moise, B. Clement, M. Raissis, and P. Nanopoulos. A test for crossing receiver operating characteristic (ROC) curves. *Communications in Statistics - Theory and Methods*, 17:1985–2003, 1988.

[176] K. Molodianovitch, D. Faraggi, and B. Reiser. Comparing the areas under two correlated ROC curves: Parametric and non-parametric approaches. *Biometrical Journal*, 48:745–757, 2006.

[177] S. Morrison. *On the evaluation of detection and prediction performance of machine learning models, with applications to medical imaging data.* PhD Dissertation, Dept of Biostatistics, Brown University School of Public Health, 2021.

[178] B.R. Mosier and L.E. Bantis. Estimation and construction of confidence intervals for biomarker cutoff-points under the shortest euclidean distance from the ROC surface to the perfection corner. *Statistics in Medicine*, 40(20):4522–4539, 2021.

[179] C. Moskowitz and M.S. Pepe. Quantifying and comparing the predictive accuracy of continuous prognostic factors for binary outcomes. *Biostatistics*, 5(1):113–127, 2004.

[180] D. Mossman. Resampling techniques in the analysis of non-binormal ROC data. *Medical Decision Making*, 15:358–366, 1995.

[181] D. Mossman. Three-way ROCs. *Medical Decision Making*, 19:78–89, 1999.

[182] S.L. Mumford, E.F. Schisterman, A. Vexler, and A. Liu. Pooling biospecimens and limits of detection: Effects on ROC curve analysis. *Biostatistics*, 7(4):585–598, 2006.

[183] C. Nakas, C.T. Yiannoutsos, R.J. Bosch, and C. Moyssiadis. Assessment of diagnostic markers by goodness-of-fit tests. *Statistics in Medicine*, 22:2503–2513, 2003.

[184] C.T. Nakas. Performance of the one-sample goodness-of-fit pp-plot length test. *Communications in Statistics - Simulation and Computation*, 36:1053–1059, 2007.

[185] C.T. Nakas. Developments in ROC surface analysis and assessment of diagnostic markers in three-class classification problems. *REVSTAT Stat J*, 12(1):43–65, 2014.

[186] C.T. Nakas and T.A. Alonzo. ROC graphs for assessing the ability of a diagnostic marker to detect three disease classes with an umbrella ordering. *Biometrics*, 63(2):603–609, 2007.

[187] C.T. Nakas, T.A. Alonzo, and C.T. Yiannoutsos. Accuracy and cut-off point selection in three-class classification problems using a generalization of the youden index. *Statistics in Medicine*, 29(28):2946–2955, 2010.

[188] C.T. Nakas, J.C. Dalrymple-Alford, T. Anderson, and T.A. Alonzo. Generalization of youden index for multiple-class classification problems applied to the assessment of externally validated cognition in parkinson disease screening. *Statistics in Medicine*, 32(6):995–1003, 2013.

[189] C.T. Nakas and B. Reiser. Editorial for the special issue of "statistical methods in medical research" on "advanced roc analysis". *Statistical Methods in Medical Research*, 27(3):649–650, 2018.

[190] C.T. Nakas and C.T. Yiannoutsos. Ordered multiple-class ROC analysis with continuous measurements. *Statistics in Medicine*, 23:3437–3449, 2004.

[191] G.J. Nehls and G.G. Akland. Procedures for handling aerometric data. *Journal for Air Pollution Control Association*, 7(8):585–598, 2006.

[192] R.G. Newcombe. Confidence intervals for an effect size measure based on the mann-whitney statistic. Part 2: Asymptotic methods and evaluation. *Statistics in Medicine*, 25:559–573, 2006.

[193] S. Noll, R. Furrer, B. Reiser, and C.T. Nakas. Inference in receiver operating characteristic surface analysis via a trinormal model-based testing approach. *Stat*, 8:e249, 2019.

[194] A.D. Nze Ossima, J.P. Daurès, F. Bessaoud, and B. Trétarre. The generalized lehmann ROC curves: Lehmann family of ROC surfaces. *Journal of Statistical Computation and Simulation*, 85:596–607, 2015.

[195] N.A. Obuchowski. Multireader, multimodality receiver operating characteristic curve studies: Hypothesis testing and sample size estimation using an analysis of variance approach with dependent observations. *Academic Radiology*, 2:S22–9, 1995.

[196] N.A. Obuchowski. Testing for equivalence of diagnostic tests. *American Journal of Roentgenology*, 168:13–17, 1997.

[197] N.A. Obuchowski. Sample size calculations in studies of test accuracy. *Statistical Methods in Medicinal Research*, 7:371–392, 1998.

[198] N.A. Obuchowski. Can electronic medical images replace hard-copy film? Defining and testing the equivalence of diagnostic tests. *Statistics in Medicine*, 20:2845–2863, 2001.

[199] N.A. Obuchowski. An ROC-type measure of diagnostic accuracy when the gold standard is continuous-scale. *Statistics in Medicine*, 25:481–493, 2006.

[200] N.A. Obuchowski and D.K. McClish. Sample size determination for diagnostic accuracy studies involving binormal ROC curve indices. *Statistics in Medicine*, 16:1529–1542, 1997.

[201] N.A. Obuchowski and H.E. Rockette. Hypothesis testing of diagnostic accuracy for multiple readers and multiple tests: An anova approach with dependent observations. *Communications in Statistics – Simulation and Computation*, 24:285–308, 1995.

[202] C.M. Otto. Valvular aortic stenosis disease severity and timing of intervention. *Journal of the American College of Cardiology*, 47(11):2141–2151, 2006.

[203] M.S. Pepe. Three approaches to regression analysis of receiver operating characteristic curves for continuous test results. *Biometrics*, 54:124–135, 1998.

[204] M.S. Pepe. *The Statistical Evaluation of Medical Tests for Classification and Prediction.* Oxford University Press, 2004.

[205] M.S. Pepe, T. Cai, and G. Longton. Combining predictors for classification using the area under the receiver operating characteristic curve. *Biometrics*, 62:221–229, 2006.

[206] S. Perez-Jaume, K. Skaltsa, N. Pallarès, and J. Carrasco. ThresholdROC: Optimum threshold estimation tools for continuous diagnostic tests in R. *Journal of Statistical Software*, 82(4):1–21, 2017.

[207] N.J. Perkins, and E.F. Schisterman and A. Vexler. Receiver operating characteristic curve inference from a sample with a limit of detection. *American Journal of Epidemiology*, 165:325–333, 2007.

[208] N.J. Perkins and E.F. Schisterman. The inconsistency of "optimal" cutpoints using two ROC based criteria. *American Journal of Epidemiology*, 163:670–675, 2006.

[209] N.J. Perkins, E.F. Schisterman, and A. Vexler. ROC curve inference for best linear combination of two biomarkers subject to limits of detection. *Biometrical Journal*, 53(3):464–476, 2011.

[210] N.J. Perkins, E.F. Schisterman, and A. Vexler. Multivariate normally distributed biomarkers subject to limits of detection and receiver operating characteristic curve inference. *Academic Radiology*, 20(7):838–846, 2013.

[211] E.D. Pisano, C. Gatsonis, E. Hendrick, M. Yaffe, J.K. Baum, S. Acharyya, E.F. Conant, L.L. Fajardo, L. Bassett, D'Orsi, C., R. Jong, and M. Rebner. Diagnostic performance of digital versus film mammography for breast-cancer screening. *New England Journal of Medicine*, 353:1773–1783, 2005.

[212] E.D. Pisano, R.E. Hendrick, M.J. Yaffe, J.K. Baum, S. Acharyya, J.B. Cormack, L.A. Hanna, E.F. Conant, L.L. Fajardo, L.W. Bassett, C.J. D'Orsi, R.A. Jong, M. Rebner, A.N. Tosteson, C.A. Gatsonis, and DMIST Investigators Group. Diagnostic accuracy of digital versus film mammography: Exploratory analysis of selected population subgroups in dmist. *Radiology*, 246(2):376–383, 2008.

[213] S.R.S. Poduri Rao. *Variance Components: Mixed Models, Methodologies and Applications.* Chapman and Hall/CRC, 1997.

[214] L. Porte, P. Legarraga, V. Vollrath, X. Aguilera, J.M. Munita, R. Araos, G. Pizarro, P. Vial, M. Iruretagoyena, S. Dittrich, and T. Weitzel. Evaluation of a novel antigen-based rapid detection test for the diagnosis of sars-cov-2 in respiratory samples. *International Journal of Infectious Diseases*, 99:328–333, 2020.

[215] J. Pouchot, A. Grasland, C. Collet, J. Coste, J.M. Esdaile, and P. Vinceneux. Reliability of tuberculin skin test measurements. *Annals of Internal Medicine*, 126:210–214, 1997.

[216] G. Qin and L. Hotilovac. Comparison of non-parametric confidence intervals for the area under the ROC curve of a continuous-scale diagnostic test. *Statistical Methods in Medical Research*, 17:207–221, 2008.

[217] J. Qin and B. Zhang. Using logistic regression procedures for estimating receiver operating characteristic curves. *Biometrika*, 90:585–596, 2003.

[218] C. Ratnasamy, D.D. Kinnamon, S.E. Lipshultz, and P. Rusconi. Associations between neurohormonal and inflammatory activation and heart failure in children. *American Heart Journal*, 155(3):527–533, 2008.

[219] B. Reiser and D. Faraggi. Confidence intervals for the generalized ROC criterion. *Biometrics*, 53:644–652, 1997.

[220] B. Reiser and I. Guttman. Statistical inference for $pr(y < x)$: The normal case. *Technometrics*, 28:253–257, 1986.

[221] X. Robin, N. Turck, A. Hainard, N. Tiberti, F. Lisacek, J.C. Sanchez, and M. Müller. pROC: An open-source package for R and S+ to analyze and compare ROC curves. *BMC Bioinformatics*, 12:77, 2011.

[222] C. Rodenberg and X.H. Zhou. ROC curve estimation when covariates affect the verification process. *Biometrics*, 56(4):1256–1262, 2000.

[223] M.X. Rodríguez-Álvarez and V. Inácio. ROCnReg: An R package for receiver operating characteristic curve inference with and without covariates. *The R Journal*, 13:525–555, 2021.

[224] M.X. Rodríguez-Álvarez, J. Roca-Pardiñas, and C. Cadarso-Suárez. ROC curve and covariates: Extending induced methodology to the nonparametric framework. *Statistics and Computing*, 21(4):483–499, 2011.

[225] M.X. Rodríguez-Álvarez, J. Roca-Pardinas, C. Cadarso-Suárez, and P.G. Tahoces. Bootstrap-based procedures for inference in nonparametric ROC regression analysis. *Statistical Methods in Medical Research*, 27(3):740–764, 2018.

[226] C.A. Roe and C.E. Metz. Dorfman-berbaum-metz method for statistical analysis of multireader, multimodality receiver operating characteristic data: Validation with computer simulation. *Academic Radiology*, 4:298–303, 1997.

[227] J.A. Roldán Nofuentes and J.D. Luna del Castillo. Em algorithm for comparing two binary diagnostic tests when not all the patients are verified. *Journal of Statistical Computation and Simulation*, 78(1):19–35, 2008.

[228] C.M. Rutter. Bootstrap estimation of diagnostic accuracy with patient-clustered data. *Academic Radiology*, 7:413–419, 2000.

[229] B. Sahiner, H.P. Chan, and L.M. Hadjiiski. Performance analysis of three-class classifiers: Properties of a 3-D ROC surface and the normalized volume under the surface for the ideal observer. *IEEE Transactions on Medical Imaging*, 27(2):215–227, 2008.

[230] B. Sahiner, W. Chen, A. Pezeshk, and N. Petrick. Semi-parametric estimation of the area under the precision-recall curve. *Proceedings of SPIE 9787, Medical Imaging*, 97870D, 2016.

[231] M. Salicru, D. Morles, M.L. Menendez, and L. Pardo. On the applications of divergence type measures in testing statistical hypotheses. *Journal of Multivariate Statistics*, 51:372–391, 1994.

[232] K. Sarafidis, Soubasi-Griva, V., K. Piretzi, A. Thomaidou, E. Agakidou, A. Taparkou, E. Diamanti, and Drossou-Agakidou, V. Diagnostic utility of elevated serum soluble triggering receptor expressed on myeloid cells (sTREM)-1 in infected neonates. *Intensive Care Medicine*, 36(5):864–868, 2010.

[233] E.F. Schisterman, D. Faraggi, and B. Reiser. Adjusting the generalized ROC curve for covariates. *Statistics in Medicine*, 23(21):3319–3331, 2003.

[234] E.F. Schisterman, D. Faraggi, B. Reiser, and M. Trevisan. Statistical inference for the area under the receiver operating characteristic curve in the presence of random measurement error. *American Journal of Epidemiology*, 154:174–179, 2001.

[235] E.F. Schisterman and N. Perkins. Confidence intervals for the youden index and corresponding optimal cut-point. *Communications in Statistics – Simulation and Computation*, 36:549–563, 2007.

[236] C.M. Schubert, S.N. Thorsen, and M.E. Oxley. The ROC manifold for classification systems. *Pattern Recognition*, 44(2):350–362, 2011.

[237] L. Schumaker. *Spline Functions: Basic Theory,* 3rd edition. Cambridge Mathematical Library, 2007.

[238] D.W. Scott. *Multivariate Density Estimation: Theory, Practice, and Visualization.* John Wiley, New York., 1992.

[239] B.K. Scurfield. Multiple-event forced-choice tasks in the theory of signal detectability. *Journal of Mathematical Psychology*, 40(3):253–269, 1996.

[240] B.K. Scurfield. Generalization of the theory of signal detectability to n-event m-dimensional forced-choice tasks. *Journal of Mathematical Psychology*, 42(1):5–31, 1998.

[241] P. Shi and L.E. Bantis. Construction of joint confidence spaces for the optimal true class fraction triplet in the ROC space using alternative biomarker cutoffs. *Biometrical Journal*, 64(6):1023–1039, 2022.

[242] S.Y. Shiu and C. Gatsonis. The predictive receiver operating characteristic curve for the joint assessment of the positive and negative predictive value. *Philosophical Transactions of the Royal Society, Series A. Math Phys Eng Sci*, 366(1874):2313–2333, 2008.

[243] S.Y. Shiu and C. Gatsonis. On ROC analysis with nonbinary reference standard. *Biometrical Journal*, 54(4):457–480, 2012.

[244] T. Sing, O. Sander, N. Beerenwinkel, and T. Lengauer. ROCR: Visualizing classifier performance in R. *Bioinformatics*, 21(20):7881, 2005.

[245] K. Skaltsa, L. Jover, and J.L. Carrasco. Estimation of the diagnostic threshold accounting for decision costs and sampling uncertainty. *Biometrical Journal*, 52:676–697, 2010.

[246] K. Skaltsa, L. Jover, D. Fuster, and J.L. Carrasco. Optimum threshold estimation based on cost function in a multistate diagnostic setting. *Statistics in Medicine*, 31(11–12):1098–1109, 2012.

[247] P. Skendros, P. Boura, D. Chrisagis, and Raptopoulou-Gigi, M. Diminished percentage of CD4+ T-lymphocytes expressing interleukine-2 receptor alpha in chronic brucellosis. *The Journal of Infection*, 54(2):192–197, 2007.

[248] E.H. Slate and B.W. Turnbull. Statistical models for longitudinal biomarkers of disease onset. *Statistics in Medicine*, 19(4):617–637, 2000.

[249] H.H. Song. Analysis of correlated ROC areas in diagnostic setting. *Biometrics*, 53:370–382, 1997.

[250] X. Song and X.H. Zhou. A semiparametric approach for the covariate specific ROC curve with survival outcome. *Statistica Sinica*, 18:947–965, 2008.

[251] A. Sorribas, J. March, and J. Trujillano. A new parametric method based on S-distributions for computing receiver operating characteristic curves for continuous diagnostic tests. *Statistics in Medicine*, 21:1213–1235, 2002.

[252] M.A. Stephens. Edf statistics for goodness of fit and some comparisons. *Journal of the American Statistical Association*, 69:730–737, 1974.

[253] E.W. Steyerberg, A.J. Vickers, N.R. Cook, T. Gerds, M. Gönen, N. Obuchowski, M.J. Pencina, and M.W. Kattan. Assessing the performance of prediction models: A framework for traditional and novel measures. *Epidemiology*, 21(1):128–138, 2010.

[254] J.Q. Su and J.S. Liu. Linear combinations of multiple diagnostic markers. *Journal of the American Statistical Association*, 88:1350–1355, 1993.

[255] J.A. Swets and R.M. Pickett. *Evaluation of Diagnostic Systems*. Academic Press, 1982.

[256] M.L. Thompson and W. Zucchini. On the statistical analysis of ROC curves. *Statistics in Medicine*, 8:1277–1290, 1989.

[257] L. Tian, C. Xiong, C.Y. Lai, and A. Vexler. Exact confidence interval estimation for the difference in diagnostic accuracy with three ordinal diagnostic groups. *Journal of Statistical Planning and Inference*, 141(1):549–558, 2011.

[258] D.-K. To. bcROCsurface: An R package for correcting verification bias in estimation of the ROC surface and its volume for continuous diagnostic tests. *BMC Bioinformatics*, 18:503, 2017.

[259] D.-K. To, G. Adimari, and M. Chiogna. Estimation of the volume under a ROC surface in presence of covariates. *Computational Statistics and Data Analysis*, 174:107434, 2022.

[260] D.-K. To, M. Chiogna, and G. Adimari. Bias-corrected methods for estimating the receiver operating characteristic surface of continuous diagnostic tests. *Electronic Journal of Statistics*, 10(2):3063–3113, 2016.

[261] D.-K. To, M. Chiogna, and G. Adimari. Nonparametric estimation of ROC surfaces under verification bias. *REVSTAT - Statistical Journal*, 18:697–720, 2020.

[262] A. Toledano and C. Gatsonis. Ordinal regression methodology for ROC curves derived from correlated data. *Statistics in Medicine*, 15:1807–1826, 1996.

[263] A. Toledano and C. Gatsonis. Missing data in ROC curve analysis. *Biometrics*, 55:488–496, 1999.

[264] A.Y. Toledano. Three methods for analysing correlated ROC curves: A comparison in real data sets from multi-reader, multi-case studies with a factorial design. *Statistics in Medicine*, 22:2919–2933, 2003.

[265] A.N.A. Tosteson and C.B. Begg. A general regression methodology for ROC curve estimation. *Medical Decision Making*, 8:204–215, 1998.

[266] T.D. Tosteson, J.P. Buonaccorsi, E. Demidenko, and W.A. Wells. Measurement error and confidence intervals for ROC curves. *Biometrical Journal*, 47:409–416, 2005.

[267] G. Tremont, G.D. Papandonatos, B. Springate, B. Huminski, M.D. McQuiggan, J. Grace, L. Frakey, and B.R. Ott. Use of the telephone-administered minnesota cognitive acuity screen to detect mild cognitive impairment. *American Journal of Alzheimer's Disease and Other Dementias*, 26(7):555–562, 2011.

[268] C.M. Umemneku Chikere, K. Wilson, S. Graziadio, L. Vale, and A.J. Allen. Diagnostic test evaluation methodology: A systematic review of methods employed to evaluate diagnostic tests in the absence of gold standard – an update. *PLoS ONE*, 14(10):e0223832, 2019.

[269] I. Unal. Defining an optimal cut-point value in ROC analysis: An alternative approach. *Computational and Mathematical Methods in Medicine*, 2017:3762651, 2017.

[270] I. Ünal and H.R. Burgut. Verification bias on sensitivity and specificity measurements in diagnostic medicine: A comparison of some approaches used for correction. *Journal of Applied Statistics*, 41(5):1091–1104, 2014.

[271] B. Van Calster, V. Van Belle, Y. Vergouwe, and E.W. Steyerberg. Discrimination ability of prediction models for ordinal outcomes: Relationships between existing measures and a new measure. *Biometrical Journal*, 54(5):674–685, 2012.

[272] B. Van Calster, Y. Vergouwe, C.W.N. Looman, V. Van Belle, D. Timmerman, and E.W. Steyerberg. Assessing the discriminative ability of risk models for more than two outcome categories. *European Journal of Epidemiology*, 27(10):761–770, 2012.

[273] A.W. van der Vaart. *Asymptotic Statistics.* Cambridge University Press, 2000.

[274] E. Venkatraman and C.B. Begg. A distribution-free procedure for comparing receiver operating characteristic curves from a paired experiment. *Biometrika*, 83:835–848, 1996.

[275] A. Vexler, A. Liu, E. Eliseeva, and E.F. Schisterman. Maximum likelihood ratio tests for comparing the discriminatory ability of biomarkers subject to limit of detection. *Biometrics*, 64(3):895–903, 2008.

[276] A.J. Vickers and E.B. Elkin. Decision curve analysis: A novel method for evaluating prediction models. *Medical Decision Making*, 26(6):565–574, 2006.

[277] A.J. Vickers, B. van Calster, and E.W. Steyerberg. Net benefit approaches to the evaluation of prediction models, molecular markers, and diagnostic tests. *BMJ*, 352(i6), 2016.

[278] A.J. Vickers, B. van Calster, and E.W. Steyerberg. A simple, step-by-step guide to interpreting decision curve analysis. *Diagnostic and Prognostic Research*, 3(18), 2019.

[279] W. Waegeman, B. De Baets, and L. Boullart. Learning layered ranking functions with structured support vector machines. *Neural Networks*, 21(10):1511–1523, 2008.

[280] W. Waegeman, B. De Baets, and L. Boullart. On the scalability of ordered multi-class ROC analysis. *Computational Statistics and Data Analysis*, 52(7):3371–3388, 2008.

[281] S.J. Walsh. Goodness-of-fit issues in ROC curve estimation. *Medical Decision Making*, 19:193–201, 1999.

[282] S. Wan. An empirical likelihood confidence interval for the volume under ROC surface. *Statistics and Probability Letters*, 82(7):1463–1467, 2012.

[283] S. Wan and B. Zhang. Semiparametric ROC surfaces for continuous diagnostic tests based on two test measurements. *Statistics in Medicine*, 28(18):2370–2383, 2009.

[284] M.P. Wand and M.C. Jones. *Kernel Smoothing.* Chapman & Hall / CRC, 1995.

[285] M.S. Wandishin and S.J. Mullen. Multiclass ROC analysis. *Weather and Forecasting*, 24(2):530–547, 2009.

[286] D. Wang, K. Attwood, and L. Tian. Receiver operating characteristic analysis under tree orderings of disease classes. *Statistics in Medicine*, 35:1907–1926, 2016.

[287] D. Wang and X. Cai. Smooth ROC curve estimation via bernstein polynomials. *PLoS ONE*, 15:e0251959, 2021.

[288] S. Wellek. *Testing Statistical Hypotheses of Equivalence and Noninferiority,* 2nd edition. CRC Press, 2010.

[289] S. Wieand, M.H. Gail, B.R. James, and K.L. James. A family of nonparametric statistics for comparing diagnostic markers with paired or unpaired data. *Biometrika*, 76:585–592, 1989.

[290] M. Wu, E. Pisano, and Y. Zheng. Information systems and health care iv: Real-time ROC analysis to evaluate radiologists' performance of interpreting mammography. *Communications of the Association for Information Systems*, doi.org/10.17705/1CAIS.01616, 2005.

[291] M. Wu, Y. Shu, Z. Li, and A. Liu. Repeated significance tests of linear combinations of sensitivity and specificity of a diagnostic biomarker. *Statistics in Medicine*, 35:3397–3412, 2016.

[292] C. Xiong, J. Luo, L. Chen, F. Gao, J. Liu, G. Wang, R. Bateman, and J.C. Morris. Estimating diagnostic accuracy for clustered ordinal diagnostic groups in the three-class case – application to the early diagnosis of alzheimer disease. *Statistical Methods in Medical Research*, 27(3):701–714, 2018.

[293] C. Xiong, G. van Belle, J.P. Miller, and J.C. Morris. Measuring and estimating diagnostic accuracy when there are three ordinal diagnostic groups. *Statistics in Medicine*, 25:1251–1273, 2006.

[294] C. Xiong, G. van Belle, J.P. Miller, Y. Yan, F. Gao, K. Yu, and J.C. Morris. A parametric comparison of diagnostic accuracy with three ordinal diagnostic groups. *Biometrical Journal*, 49(5):682–693, 2007.

[295] Q. Yan, L.E. Bantis, J.L. Stanford, and Z. Feng. Combining multiple biomarkers linearly to maximize the partial area under the ROC curve. *Statistics in Medicine*, 37:627–642, 2018.

[296] H. Yang and D. Carlin. ROC surface: A generalization of ROC curve analysis. *Journal of Biopharmaceutical Statistics*, 10(2):183–196, 2000.

[297] H. Yang and L. Zhao. A method of estimating and comparing volumes under receiver operating characteristic (ROC) surfaces. *Statistics in Biopharmaceutical Research*, 2(2):279–291, 2010.

[298] F. Yao, R.V. Craiu, and B. Reiser. Nonparametric covariate adjustment for receiver operating characteristic curves. *The Canadian Journal of Statistics*, 38(1):27–46, 2010.

[299] C.T. Yiannoutsos, C.T. Nakas, and B.A. Navia. Assessing multiple-group diagnostic problems with multi-dimensional receiver operating characteristic surfaces: Application to proton mr spectroscopy (mrs) in hiv-related neurological injury. *Neuroimage*, 40(1):248–255, 2008.

[300] J. Yin, C.T. Nakas, L. Tian, and B. Reiser. Confidence intervals for differences between volumes under receiver operating characteristic surfaces (vus) and generalized youden indices (gyis). *Statistical Methods in Medical Research*, 27:675–688, 2018.

[301] J. Yin and L. Tian. Optimal linear combinations of multiple diagnostic biomarkers based on youden index. *Statistics in Medicine*, 33:1426–1440, 2014.

[302] W.J. Youden. Index for rating diagnostic tests. *Cancer*, 3:32–35, 1950.

[303] T. Yu. ROCs: Receiver operating characteristic surface for class-skewed high-throughput data. *PLoS ONE*, 7(7):at. no. e40598, 2012.

[304] Y. Zhang and T.A. Alonzo. Estimation of the volume under the receiver-operating characteristic surface adjusting for non-ignorable verification bias. *Statistical Methods in Medical Research*, 27(3):715–739, 2018.

[305] Z. Zhang and Y. Huang. A linear regression framework for the receiver operating characteristic (ROC) curve analysis. *Journal of Biometrics & Biostatistics*, 3(2), 2005.

[306] Y. Zheng and P.J. Heagerty. Semiparametric estimation of time-dependent ROC curves for longitudinal marker data. *Biostatistics*, 5(4):615–632, 2004.

[307] H. Zhou and G. Qin. Confidence intervals for the difference in paired youden indices. *Pharmaceutical Statistics*, 12:17–27, 2013.

[308] X.H. Zhou. Maximum likelihood estimators of sensitivity and specificity corrected for verification bias. *Communications in Statistics – Theory and Methods*, 22(11):3177–3198, 1993.

[309] X.H. Zhou. Effect of verification bias on positive and negative predictive values. *Statistics in Medicine*, 13(17):1737–1745, 1994.

[310] X.H. Zhou. Comparing accuracies of two screening tests in a two-phase study for dementia. *Journal of the Royal Statistical Society: Series C (Applied Statistics)*, 47(1):135–147, 1998.

[311] X.H. Zhou, P. Castellucio, and C. Zhou. Nonparametric estimation of ROC curves in the absence of a gold standard. *Biometrics*, 61:600–609, 2001.

[312] X.H. Zhou and C.A. Gatsonis. A simple method for comparing correlated ROC curves using incomplete data. *Statistics in Medicine*, 15:1687–1693, 1996.

[313] X.H. Zhou and J. Harezlak. Comparison of bandwidth selection methods for kernel smoothing of ROC curves. *Statistics in Medicine*, 21:2045–2055, 2002.

[314] X.H. Zhou, N.A. Obuchowski, and D.K. McClish. *Statistical Methods in Diagnostic Medicine,* 2nd edition. Wiley Interscience, 2011.

[315] G.Y. Zou and L. Yue. Using confidence intervals to compare several correlated areas under the receiver operating characteristic curves. *Statistics in Medicine*, 32:5077–5090, 2013.

[316] K.H. Zou, W. Hall, and D.E. Shapiro. Smooth non-parametric receiver operating characteristic curves for continuous diagnostic tests. *Statistics in Medicine*, 16:2143–2156, 1997.

[317] K.H. Zou and W.J. Hall. Two transformation models for estimating an ROC curve from continuous data. *Journal of Applied Statistics*, 27: 621–631, 2000.

[318] K.H. Zou, A. Liu, A.I. Bandos, L. Ohno-Machado, and H. Rockette. *Statistical Evaluation of Diagnostic Performance Topics in ROC Analysis.* CRC Press, 2012.

Index

Note: Locators in *italics* represent figures and **bold** indicate tables in the text.

A

acc_cca function, 166
Acceptance radius, 33
Accuracy, 1, 2
Akritas, M. G., 157
Alonzo, T. A., 94, 127, 129, 136, 168, 169, 171
Area under the ROC curve (AUC), 3, 11, 23, 27–29
Arifin, W. N., 164, 167, 168
Arterial stenosis, 2
Asymptotic integrated mean squared error (AMISE), 99

B

Bamber, D., 168
Bandos, A. I., 33, 94
Bantis, L. E., 31, 34, 68, 80, 82, 96–98, 104, 125–126, 131, 133–134, 136, 143–144, 174–175, 177
Begg and Greenes method (BG), 166–167
Begg, C. B., 103, 104, 138, 164, 166, 182
Bernstein polynomials, 69
Binary disease status, 5, 35
Binary logistic regression model, 150, 152
Binary-scaled marker, 23, 43–44, **44**
Binary tests
- confusion matrix, 19, 21, **21**
- cross classification, **18**
- diagnostic and predictive accuracy, **20**
- diagnostic performance, 18–19, 22–24
- overall accuracy and error rate, 19
- predictive performance, 18

Binomial distribution theory, 21
Binormal model, 146–148
- Box-Cox transformation, 51–54, *53*
- continuous marker measurements, 57
- improper and proper, 49
- intercept and slope of curves, 48
- ordinal marker measurements, 54–57, **56**
- parameters, 48, *49*
- pointwise confidence bands, 58–59
- role of, 48

Blackwelder, W. C., 105
Bootstrap, 64, 67, 77, *82*, 94–95
Bootstrap-based inference, 64, 74
Box-Cox transformation, 51–54, *53*, 89, 91, 92, 98, 104, 115, 116, 125–126, 132
Branscum, A. J., 69
Braun, T. M., 94
Brucellosis, 7–8, *9*, 39, 76, 107
Brumback, L. C., 143

C

Cai, T., 142, 158
Carlin, D., 136
CD3 T-lymphocytes, 8
CD4 T-lymphocytes, 8

Coffin, M., 178
Complete case approach (CCA), 165
Complex designs
correlated ordinal categorical data, 153–154
hierarchical ROC analysis, 154
Jackknife and bootstrap methods, 154–155
sample size considerations, 155–156
Conditional distribution, 2
Conditional independence assumption (CIA), 180, 182, 183
Conditional probability, 2–3, 6, 19
Confidence intervals, 80, 94, 133
Confusion matrix, 19, 21, **21**
Continuous-scaled (CD4) markers, 39–42, *40, 41*, 69–70, 104
Coronary artery disease (CAD), 164
Cox regression models, 142–143
c-statistics, 3
Cumulative distribution functions (CDF) plots, 3, *4*
Cut-off points
Euclidean distance, 133–135, *134, 135*
generalized Youden index, 131–133
sensitivity and specificity, 81–82

D

Data sets
CD3, CD4 data, 8
mammography data, 11, 14–15
pancreatic cancer data, **12**
Parkinson Disease data, **13**
Decision curve analysis, 34
De Long, E. R., 71, 83, 95, 103
Delta method, 48, 57, 59, 72, 73, 77–79, *82*, 83, 87, 96, 100, 120, 123, 124, 126, 179
Descriptive statistics, 7–10, **8, 12–13**
Diagnostic accuracy, 1, 3
Digital Mammography Imaging Screening Trial (DMIST), 10–11, 22, 37, 38, **43**, 55, 87, 138
Doubly robust (DR) estimators, 169

E

Elkin, E. B., 34
Empirical PROC curve, 36
Empirical ROC curves
absence of ties, 25, **26**, 28
hypothesis testing, 62
marker values, 24
presence of ties, 25, **26**, *27*, **27**
sensitivity and specificity, 60
Equivalence assessment, 105
Euclidean-based cut-offs, 133–135, *134, 135*
Extended Begg and Greens (EBG) method, 166
Extended generalized gamma (EGG) model, 175, 177

F

False Class Fractions (FCF), 113
False negative rate, **18**
False positive rate, **18**
Faraggi, D., 144, 177,
Feng, Z., 97, 104, 125, 126, 136
F, F_1 score, 20
Finite Polya Tree (FPT) hierarchical prior distributions, 115
Free-Response ROC analysis (FROC), 33
Full-field digital mammography (FFDM), 11
Full imputation (FI) method, 168, 171
Fundamental property of diagnostic tests, 3

G

Gatsonis, C. A., 35, 36, 95, 136, 138, 154
Gaussian Kernel estimation, 64, 65, *66*

Generalized Estimating Equations (GEE), 153
Generalized ROC (gROC), 33–34, *35*
Generalized Youden index, 7, 130–135
Greenes, R. A., 164, 166, 167
Guttman, I., 73

H
Hall, P., 69
Hall, W. J., 51, 57
Hanson, T. E., 69
Harezlak, J., 64
Hazard Constrained Natural Spline (HCNS), 67
Heagerty, P. J., 156, 158, 159
Hierarchical ROC analysis, 154
Histograms, 3, *4*, 26, *28*
Hotilovac, L., 72
Huang, Y., 144
Hui, S. L., 182
Hypervolume Under the ROC hypersurface (HUR), 130

I
Ignorance region, 164
Imaging technologies, 1
Imperfect reference standard bias
  binary markers, 180–182, **181**
  description, 179–180
  non-binary markers, 182–183
  tests, 179
Improper ROC curves, 31
Inácio de Carvalho, V., 136, 144
Incomplete gamma function, 176
Interleukin-6 (IL-6), 8
Inverse cumulative distribution function (ICDF), 24
Inverse probability weighting (IPW) approach, 168–171
Ishwaran, H., 154

J
Jackknife and bootstrap methods, 154–155
Jones, M. C., 63
Joseph, L., 182

K
Kaplan-Meier (KM) estimator, 69, 157
k-class ROC, 135–136
Kernel-based estimators, 31, 177
Kernel density estimation, 63, 99, 131
K-nearest neighbor (KNN), 171
Kolmogorov-Smirnov (KS) two-sample statistics, 62

L
LABROC4 program, 57, 69
Late-onset sepsis (LOS), 8, 88–89, 93, 95, 103
Length of ROC curve, 31–32
Likelihood ratio, positive, negative, **20**
Limit of detection (LoD)
  Box-Cox and extended generalized gamma ROC curves, 175–177, *176*
  defined, 174
  empirical ROC, 174–175
  hybrid approach, 177
  maximum likelihood ratio tests, 174
  ROC analysis framework, 174
Location parameter vector, 54, 138
Location-scale models, 141–142
Logspline survival function, 67

M
Machine learning, 19, 145–146
Ma, G., 57
Mammography data, 11, 14–15
Mann-Whitney statistics, 29
Mantoux skin test, 180
Margin of equivalence, 105
Matsui, S., 145
McClish, D. K., 81, 106, 107

Mean score imputation (MSI) approach, 168, 170–171
Measurement error
  confidence interval, 173, 177–178
  error/variability, 177
  parametric analysis, 178–179
Metropolis–Hastings algorithm, 118
Metz, C. E., 57–58, 69, 83, 92, 100, 104, 122, 182
Mini Mental State Examination (S-MMSE), 9
Missing at random (MAR), 162
Missing completely at random (MCAR), 162
Missing not at random (MNAR), 166
Moise, A., 94
Montreal Cognitive Assessment test (MoCA), 9
Mossman, D., 94, 135
Multinomial logistic regression model, 170, 172
Multi-reader, multi-case (MRMC) studies, 155–156

N

Nakas, C., 62, 112, 114, 127, 129, 130, 135, 136
Negative predictive value (NPV), 2–3, 6, 18–19, **20**, 35, 36, 163
Net benefit approach, 34
Newcombe, R. G., 72
Noll, S., 48, 122
Non-binary markers, 23, 182–183
Non-inferiority assessment, 105
Nonparametric AUC comparisons
  bootstrap, 94–95
  U-statistics, 93–94
Nonparametric method, 37
  AUC, 71–72
  Kernel-based ROCs, 63–66
  spline-based ROCs, 66–70
Nze Ossima, A. D., 144

O

Obuchowski, N. A., 33, 105–107, 130
Omnibus comparisons
  nonparametric method, 103–104
  parametric methods, 100–103
Ordinal categorical markers, 87, 139
Ordinal-scaled marker, 42, *43*, 95
Overall accuracy, 2

P

"Paired" designs, 86
Pancreatic cancer data, 109, 120, 140, 145, 147, 150, 152
Parametric AUC comparisons
  binormal model, 92
  normally distributed, continuous test data, 87–89
  ordinal categorical test data, 87
Parametric methods, 37, 72–74
Parkinson disease (PD) data, 9–10
Partial Area under the ROC Curve (pAUC), 27, 28
  statistical inference, 77–78
PD patients either with dementia (PD-D), 57
PD patients either with mild cognitive impairment (PD-MCI), 57
Pearson correlation coefficients, 124
Pepe, M. S., 36, 144, 163, 168, 169, 171
Perkins, N. J., 30, 59, 79, 97, 174–175
Permutation tests, 76, 94
Point-closest-to-(0,1) approach, 30
Porte, L., 43
Positive predictive value (PPV), 2–3, 6, 19, **20**, 36
Positron Emission Tomography (PET), 2
Pouchot, J., 180
Precision, 2, **20**
Precision-Recall (PR) curve, 36–38, *37*
Predictive accuracy, 1–2

Predictive ROC curve (PROC), 4, 34–36

Q
Qin, G., 72, 96
Quasi-likelihood, 141

R
Randomization tests, 31
Random measurement error, 177–178
Reader study, 138
Regression models for ROC analysis
 biomarker scores, 138
 computations, 140–141, *141*
 continuous markers, 139–140
 diagnostic performance, 138
 DMIST trial, 138
 parametric methods
  computations, 140–141
  continuous markers, 139–140
  ordinal categorical markers, 139
 semi-parametric methods
  Cox regression models, 142–143
  location-scale models, 141–142
Reiser, B., 73, 136
Robin, X., 94
ROC curves; *see also* Complex designs; Imperfect reference standard bias; Measurement error
 asbio package in R, *45*
 curve evaluation after logistic regression, 150–153
 definition, 23–24
 empirical, *see* Empirical ROC curves
 essentials, 32
 length of, 31
 omnibus comparisons, *see* Omnibus comparisons
 sample sizes, 105–108
 screen-film imaging, breast cancer, *43*
ROCFIT program, 183
ROC surface
 defined, 112
 empirical and general nonparametric estimation, 114–115
 hypersurfaces, multiple-class classification, 129–130
 parametric estimation, 114–115
 umbrella/tree orderings, 127–129
Rodriguez-Alvarez, M. X., 144
Rutter, C. M., 94

S
Sample size considerations
 single AUC, 104–105
 comparison of two AUCÕs, 92, 93
Sarafidis, K., 8, 10
Scale parameter vector, 54, 138
Schisterman, E. F., 30, 59, 79, 97, 144, 178–179
Scott, D. W., 99
Scurfield, B. K., 135
Semiparametric efficient (SPE), 171
Sensitivity, 2, 3, 19
Sensitivity-Specificity trade-off, 3
Shapiro-Wilk normality test, **8, 10, 12, 13**
Shi, P., 136
Shiu, S. Y., 36, 136
Single-photon-emission computed-tomography (SPECT), 164, 165
Single-point summaries, 5
Skaltsa, K., 30, 131
Skendros, P., 7–8
Slate, E. H., 158
Soluble triggering receptor expressed on myeloid cells-1 (sTREM-1), 8, **10, 11**, 52, 88, 91, 92
Specificity, 2, 3, 19
Standard Uptake Value (SUV), 2

Sukhatme, S., 178
Symbolic programming, 73

T
Target condition, 2
TB skin test, 180
Technology assessment, 4, 86, 108
Test results, 1–2
Three-class (ROC surface) analysis
  implementation using R, 171–173
  reference standard process, 168
  verified individuals, 170
Three-class model, 112–114
Tian, L., 115, 116, 119, 122, 136, 145
Time-dependent ROC analysis, 3, 6
  cumulative/dynamic, 157–158
  estimation, 157
  incident/dynamic, 159
  incident/static, 158
  sensitivity and specificity, 156–157
To, D. -K., 144, 170, 171
Toledano, A., 138
Tosteson, A. N. A., 138
Tosteson, T. D., 179
Trinormal model, 115–118, *116*
trinROC package, 112
True class fractions (TCF), 113
True negative rate, 2, **20**
True positive rate, 2, **20**
Tsimikas, J. V., 131
Turnbull, B. W., 62, 144, 158

U
Umemneku Chikere, C. M., 162
Unal, I., 80
U-statistics theory, 71, 77, 94, 119

V
Van Calster, B., 119
Venkatraman, E., 103
Verification bias
  binary test evaluation, 162–164, **163**
  defined, 161
  mechanisms, 162
  ROC curve estimation, 168–169
  subjects/subgroups, 161
Vickers, A. J., 34
Volume Under the ROC Surface (VUS), 7, 112, 116, 118–119
  comparing two markers, 121–122
  defined, 118
  diagnostic markers, 121–122
  hypothesis testing, 119–120
  parametric estimation, 119
  single marker assessment, 126–127

W
Wald confidence intervals, 166
Wand, M. P., 63
Wang, D., 129
Wan, S., 119, 136
Wieand, S., 87, 89
Wilcoxon-Mann-Whitney statistics, 71, 106, 135

X
Xiong, C., 120, 122, 130, 135, 136

Y
Yang, H., 136
Yan, Q., 145, 148, 149
Yao, F., 144
Yiannoutsos, C. T., 114, 129, 135
Yin, J., 132, 136, 145
Youden index; *see also* Cut-off points
  biomarker combinations, 148–150, *149*
  maximum of, 29–30, 70
  normally distributed marker data, 96–97
  optimal points and cut-offs, 78–81
  without normality assumption, 98
Yue, L., 93
Yusof, U. K., 164, 167

Z

Zhang, B., 136
Zhang, Y., 136
Zhang, Z., 144
Zhao, L., 136
Zheng, Y., 158, 159
Zhou, H., 96
Zhou, X. H., 64, 71, 95, 105, 140, 144, 155, 163, 164, 168, 180, 182, 183
Zou, G. Y., 93
Zou, K. H., 30, 51, 61, 63, 64, 145

Printed in the United States
by Baker & Taylor Publisher Services